A COMPLETE GUIDE TO
SLEEP SOLUTIONS

CHRIS MARSHALL

Published in 2001 by Caxton Editions
20 Bloomsbury Street
London WC1B 3JH
a member of the Caxton Publishing Group

© 2001 Caxton Publishing Group
Reprint 2002
Designed and produced for Caxton Editions
by Open Door Limited
Rutland, United Kingdom

Editing: Mary Morton
Coordination and Typesetting: Jane Booth
Digital Imagery © copyright 2001 PhotoDisc, Inc.

Title: SLEEP SOLUTIONS
ISBN: 1-84067-342-7

IMPORTANT NOTICE

This book is not intended to be a substitute for medical advice or treatment. Any
person with a condition requiring medical attention should consult a qualified
medical practitioner or suitable therapist.

A COMPLETE GUIDE TO
SLEEP SOLUTIONS

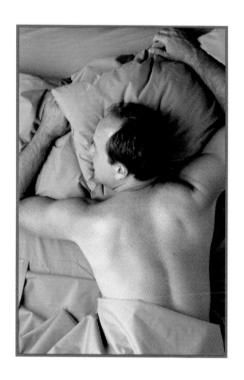

CHRIS MARSHALL

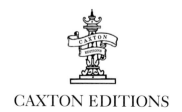

CAXTON EDITIONS

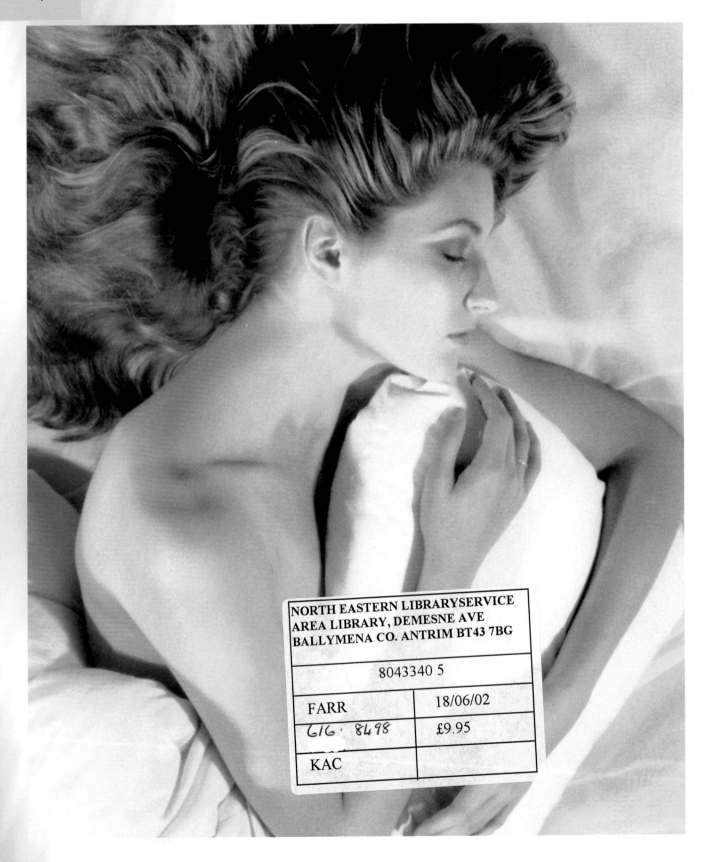

CONTENTS

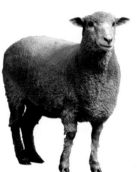

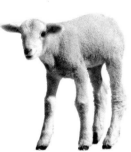

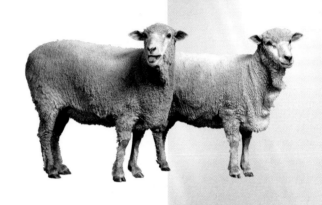

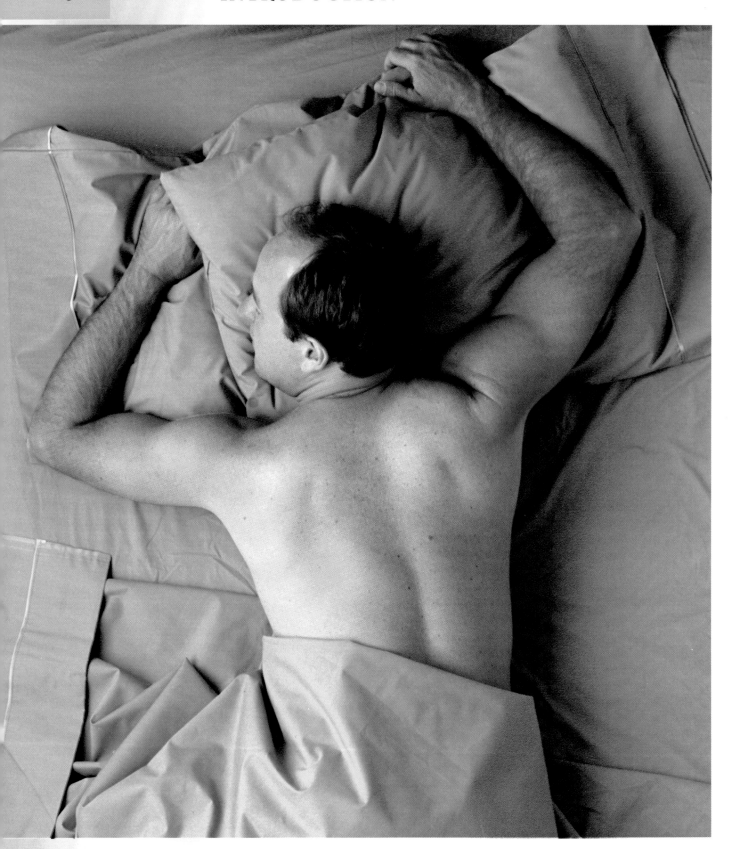

Sleep is a process that all animals and humans go through as one of the natural rhythms of life. Many people give the subject little more thought than that until a sudden bout of nightmares or insomnia disturbs this otherwise normal process. Then, suddenly, we are thrown into the twilight world of sleeplessness and begin to understand the pain and suffering that disrupted sleep can cause.

In noisy, polluted industrial countries, sleep problems are on the increase. People are crying out for sleep solutions and yet we are only just beginning to understand this most mysterious and necessary process. This book explores what is known about the purpose and nature of sleep. It also offers advice and techniques from around the world to those suffering from disrupted sleep.

Left: sleep is a process that all animals and humans go through as one of the natural rhythms of life.

Below: in noisy, polluted industrial countries sleep problems are on the increase.

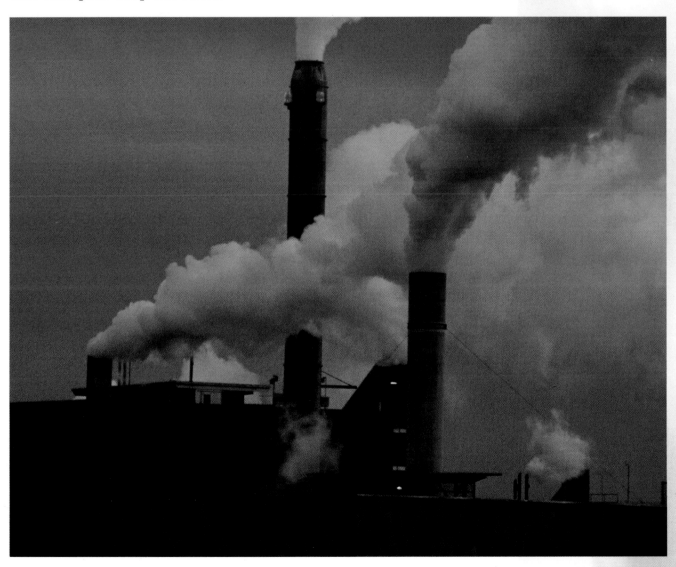

ALL ABOUT SLEEP

WHAT EXACTLY IS SLEEP?

On average, every one of us spends up to a third of our lives sleeping. As newborn babies, the average human can sleep intermittently for as long as 16 hours. By the time we are adults, we can spend between six and nine continuous hours every night in this recumbent state. But what is sleep and why do we need it? For something so familiar to all of us, the exact nature of our sleeping state is a strangely mysterious and indefinable process. It is something that has fascinated mystics, artists, philosophers and scientists alike for thousands of years.

Most of us look forward to being asleep. We see it as a welcome respite from everyday worries and activity. We relish the journey into unconsciousness and the dream state. But there are others who resent what they see as an intrusion into their waking activities. Some people even fear and dread their nightly sojourn into the altered state of sleep as their dreams take them on journeys and adventures that are wholly unwelcome. Some even worry that they may never wake up again. Then there are others who lie tossing and turning for hour after hour, feeling more and more exhausted. No matter how determined or how hard they pray for sleep, it never comes. They are unable to drift off into the regenerative slumber they need.

Below: most of us look forward to being asleep.

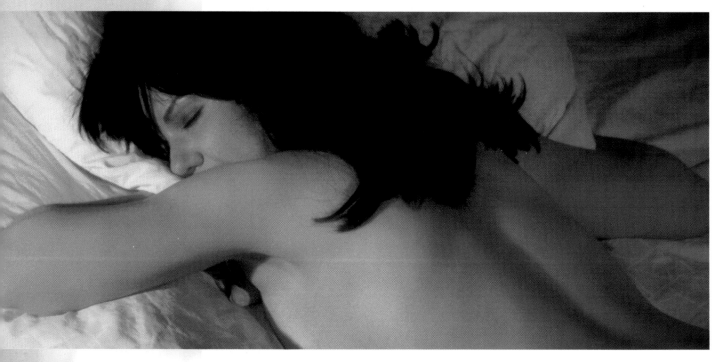

The ancient Greeks called the god of sleep Hypnos from which we derive our term for hypnotism. Hypnos was said to live in a dark cave and was the son of Nyx or night and the brother of Thanatos or death. Comparisons have often been drawn between the sleep state and death. We associate life with warmth, movement and consciousness and when we sleep, we give up this consciousness, our body temperature drops and our movements are restricted. We are somehow somewhere else. We don't really know what happens to our consciousness.

In Islam, sleep is often referred to as "the little death" and even Shakespeare referred to "that sleep of death". As humans, we have always sensed some connection between the sleeping and death state. But it is because the sleep state is such a temporary one that it fascinates us so much. We feel that if we could somehow understand what happens to us when we are asleep, we could unravel a whole lot more of the mystery of being human.

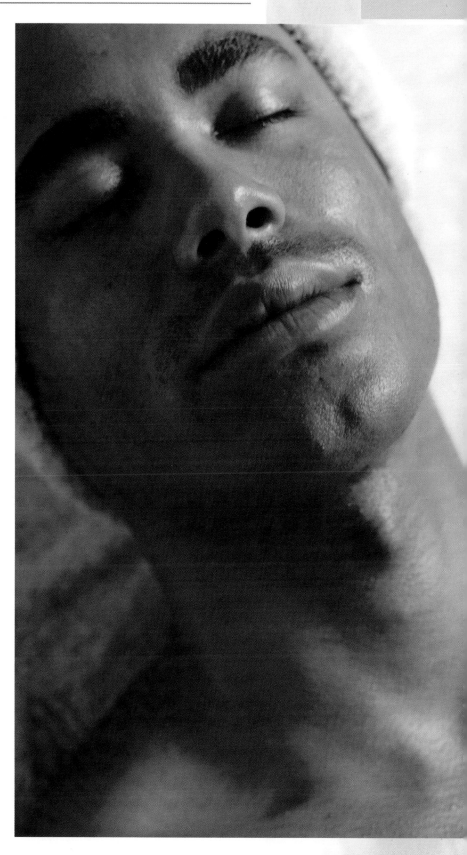

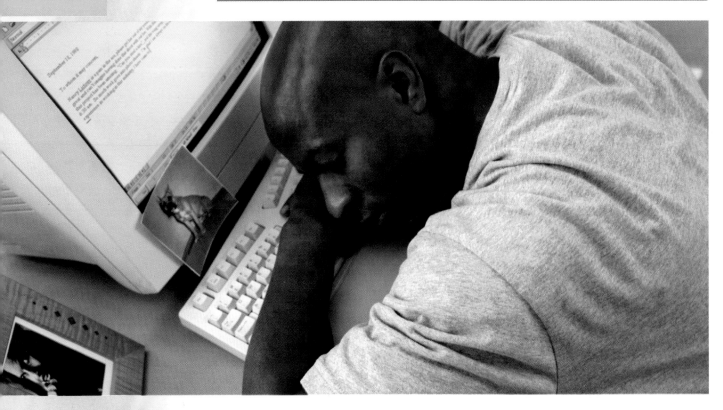

Above: some people can fall asleep in the middle of an activity.

Sleep is generally defined as that regular and recurring suspension of consciousness that provides needed rest and recuperation. It is different from coma and hibernation in that sleep is relatively spontaneous given a comfortable bed and low lighting and is easy for most of us to be woken from. But it is when we try to become specific that sleep becomes hard to define. For instance, we tend to regard sleep as something we do lying down with our eyes shut, but this is not always the case. Some people sleepwalk while others can fall asleep in the middle of an activity like driving a car with tragic consequences

One breakthrough in defining sleep was made when the German psychiatrist Hans Berger invented the electroencephalogram (EEG) in 1929. This machine measured different states of alertness. Hans Berger placed electrodes on a sleeping subject's scalp and recorded the electrical activity of their brain. This was shown as a wave on a graph and revealed how their brain activity changed whilst they were asleep.

In 1953 the psychologists Nathaniel Kleitman and his student Eugene Aserinsky used this EEG machine to demonstrate how a sleeping subject's brain activity became surprisingly similar to that of a waking person after only about an hour of sleep. During this stage, though the subject is asleep, there are rapid movements of the eyes under the eyelids. More intriguingly, if the subject was woken up while this was occurring, they reported particularly vivid memories of dreams. This phase of sleep has become known as rapid eye movement sleep or REM. A whole industry studying brain activity has grown on the back of this discovery, but the results are still far from conclusive. The exact purpose and definition of sleep remains as elusive and controversial as ever, but what has been proved is that the brain is anything but inactive during sleep.

Below: the brain is anything but inactive during sleep. There are rapid movements of the eyes under the eyelids.

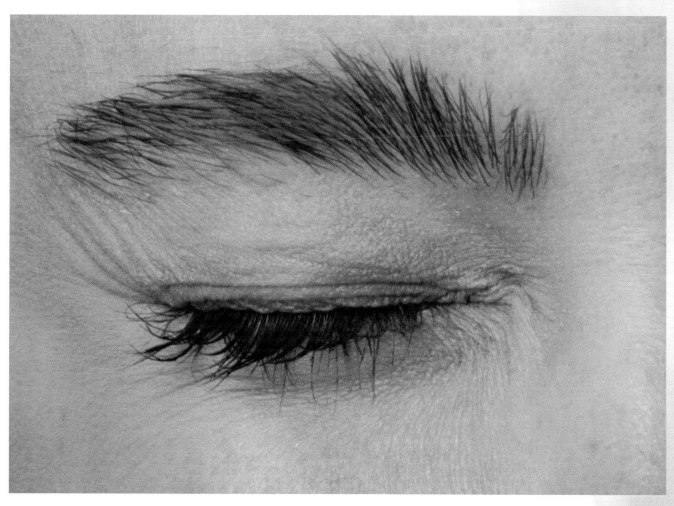

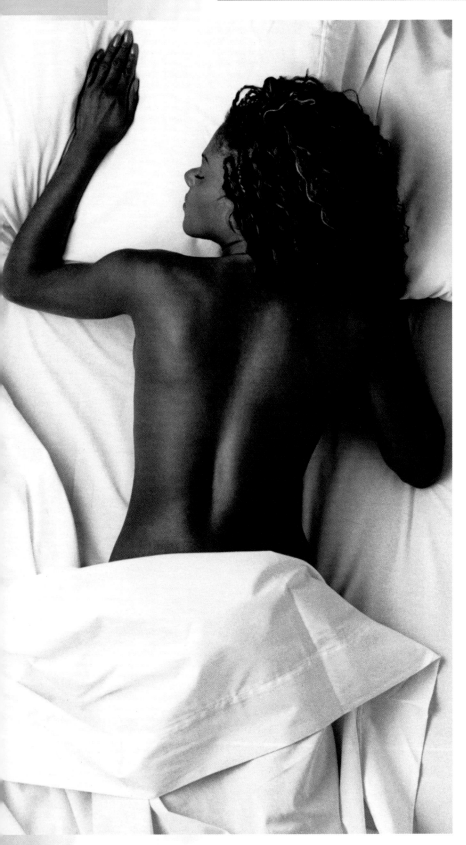

It is now understood that an average full night's sleep for an adult human is composed of several cycles each containing several stages:

Stage 1 is a period of shallow sleep during which the body temperature begins to drop. EEG readings show regular wavy lines with small undulations that suggest mental relaxation.

Stage 2 is a deeper period of sleep during which an EEG will record bursts of brain activity lasting one or two seconds known as "sleep spindles".

Stage 3 is still deeper sleep, producing large, slow waves with high voltage EEG readings that are called delta waves. 20 to 50 per cent of the brain waves are of these large, slow type.

Stage 4 is the deepest form of sleep when the brain produces over 50 per cent delta-wave activity.

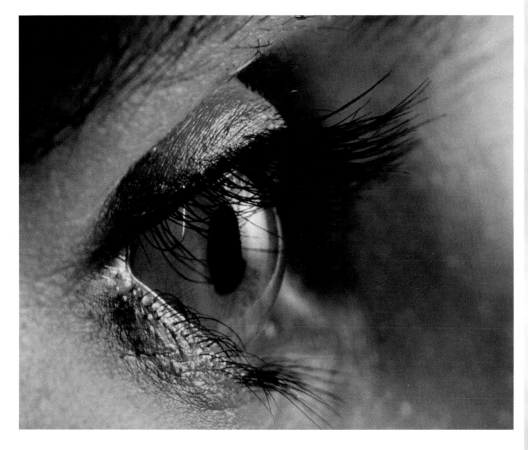

Far left: a full night's sleep for an adult is composed of several cycles.

Left: rapid eye movement sleep will account for one quarter of the sleeping time.

After Stage 4, the brain returns to Stage 3 followed by another bout of Stage 2. All of this lasts between 70 and 90 minutes and is called NREM sleep – meaning no rapid eye movement. In this NREM phase, the breathing and heart rate slows down, lowering the blood pressure. This produces a restful state during which the body recuperates and recharges.

Next comes the first bout of REM sleep lasting about ten to 15 minutes. During REM sleep, the breathing, heart rate and blood pressure all rise again and fluctuate rapidly. A near paralysis is temporarily experienced in the muscles. This is thought to be the body's way of ensuring we do not act out our dreams.

Then the whole cycle repeats again only this time, Stages 3 and 4 reduce in length while the period of REM sleep increases. During an average full night's sleep, the sleeper will go through four or five of these cycles. Rapid eye movement sleep will account for one quarter of the sleeping time while Stage 2 of deep sleep makes up most of the remaining time.

WHY DO I NEED SLEEP?

Sleep is as natural and as vital to our lives as eating and breathing – without it there can be no life. We have all had experience of disruptions to our sleeping pattern – our quality and enjoyment of life is substantially reduced within days. This fact is so obvious that sleep deprivation has long been used as a method of breaking an individual's spirit and confusing their sense of self-identity.

All living things go through periods of sleep as well as periods of wakefulness. Because it is difficult to define exactly what sleep is, it is also hard to say why we need it. It is presumed that NREM sleep gives the body an opportunity to recuperate and repair itself in preparation for the rigours of the day to come – but this has not been proved conclusively. Whilst the body certainly needs periods of rest as well as exercise, brain tissue itself does not tire in the same way that the rest of the body does. Why then do we need these nightly bouts of unconsciousness?

Below: sleep is as natural and as vital to our lives as eating and breathing.

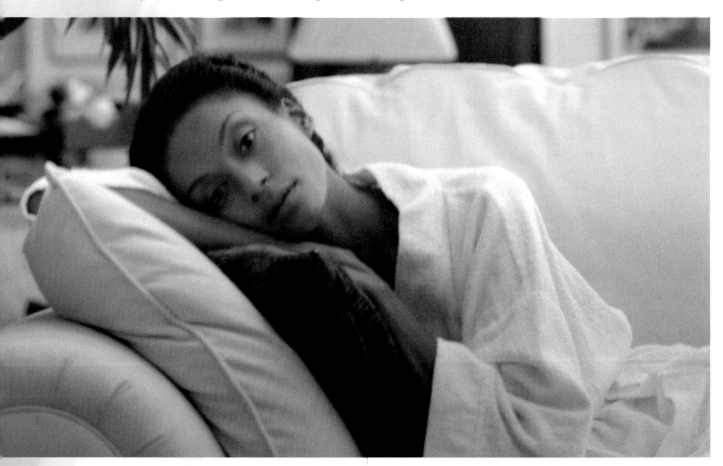

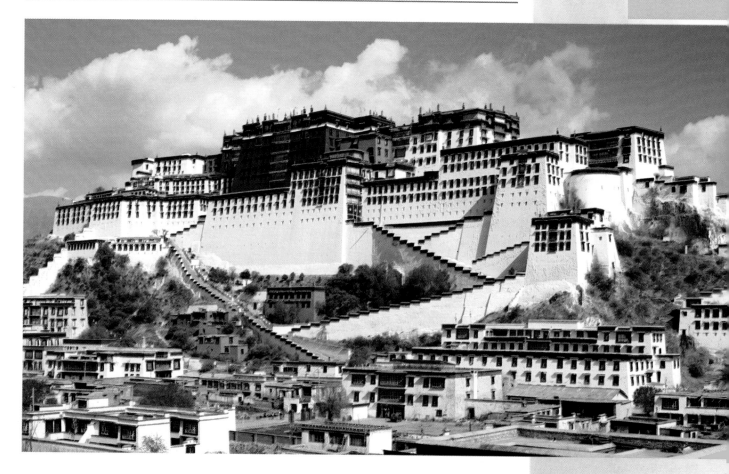

Since the body can be rested without actually sleeping and the brain itself does not get tired, perhaps we need the experience of dreaming in REM sleep. Ancient civilisations as well as many contemporary cultures regard dreaming as the time when the soul temporarily leaves the body in order to commune with the gods and spirits or other planes of consciousness. Native American Indians believe the dream state to be as real and important as any waking condition. The Australian Aboriginals consider their whole life to be a dream. The Tibetan Buddhists say that sleep takes us to those realms we all return to after death and before rebirth. The Tibetan Book of the Dead was written as advice to people of what to expect when they died. It warned that many do not realise when they have died and consider themselves to still be asleep. So in their terms, the death experience, so feared in the western world, is actually quite familiar to all of us as the place we visit every night! If this is so, then the dream state is as real and necessary to our well-being as our conscious waking experience.

Above: Buddhists say that sleep takes us to those realms we all return to after death and before rebirth.

But there are other schools of thought. Aristotle in the 4th century BC believed that dreams were little more than memories and sensory impressions distorted through the brain. In 1900 Sigmund Freud instigated a new industry by claiming dreams were the disguised expression of our unconscious desires – by and large mainly sexual – that are repressed by the conscious mind. These then spilled out as symbolic dream images.

One thing is for certain and that is that a lack of sleep has adverse effects that we are all familiar with. It is reckoned that nearly 50 per cent of all accidents are caused by a lack of quality sleep. People who sleep well generally live longer and are far healthier than those who experience long-term sleep problems. After even one night of inadequate sleep, we wake up feeling not just fatigued but irritable. We are likely to feel less inspired by life and be less productive as a consequence. Our short-term memory is impaired and our judgment feels somewhat compromised. Long-term sleep difficulties will multiply all of these problems immeasurably. Chronic insomnia will cause depression and anxiety. As the individual's stress level escalates, it becomes a Catch 22 situation. It is even harder for the sufferer to relax enough to get to sleep and a vicious circle becomes established which can lead to paranoia and other, deeper psychological problems. Long-term lack of sleep also reduces the sufferer's resistance to disease and slows down recovery from illness as the body's defence systems are undermined. Shakespeare called sleep, "the chief nourisher of life's feast". Without adequate sleep, our bodily systems starve.

Below: after even one night of inadequate sleep, we wake up feeling not just fatigued but irritable.

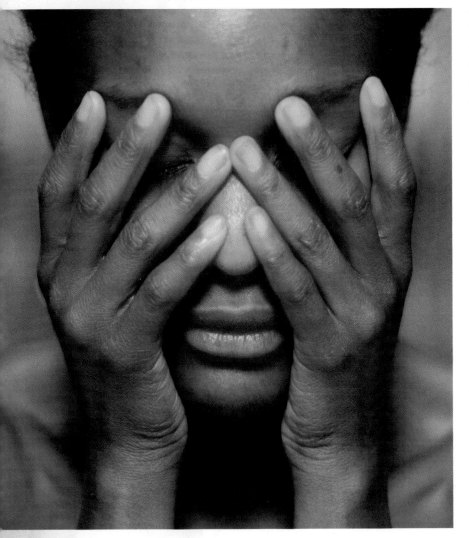

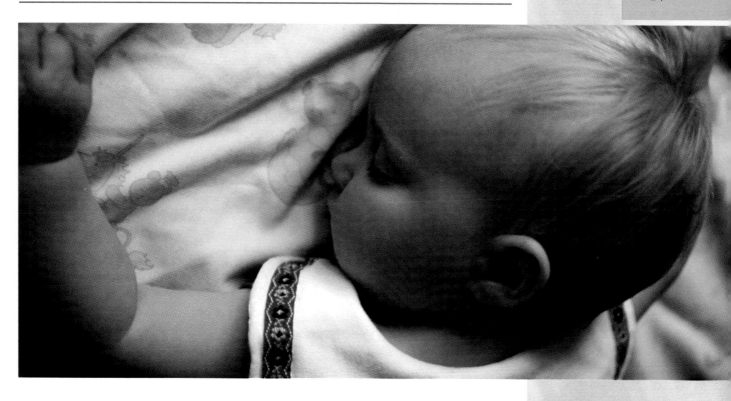

HOW MUCH SLEEP DO I NEED?

In general, each of us spends up to a third of our lives asleep. This amounts to about 25 years of slumbering in an average life span. Adults usually need between six and nine hours of sleep in every 24-hour cycle, but this naturally varies with each individual. The depth and quality of the sleep experienced must also be taken into account if comparisons are to be made. Different people need different amounts of sleep and this can vary dramatically at different stages in your life.

Babies typically will sleep between 14 and 16 hours out of every 24 though unfortunately not in a continuous stretch, as every long-suffering parent knows. Unlike adults, babies seem to bypass NREM sleep and slip straight from wakefulness into REM sleep (known as active sleep in this age group). As they grow older, babies sleep less but for longer periods at a time. By the age of three or four, young children have about three to four hours of REM sleep every 24 hours interspaced with about three hours of deep sleep and up to five hours of light sleep.

Above: babies typically will sleep between 14 and 16 hours of every 24.

Below: children between the ages of five and 15 generally need about nine hours of sleep a night.

Children between the ages of five and 15 generally need about nine hours of sleep a night.

During the formative years of adolescence, the need for sleep actually increases again and an adolescent may require about 11 hours of sleep regardless of what is on the television or what parties are on offer!

Between the ages of 20 and 30, our sleep patterns stabilise. In fact, by the time most of us are 20 years old, we average around seven and a half hours of sleep a night of which about two hours is composed of REM sleep.

By the age of around 40 to 45 in men and 50 to 55 in women, sleep patterns begin to change again although the average is still around eight hours every night.

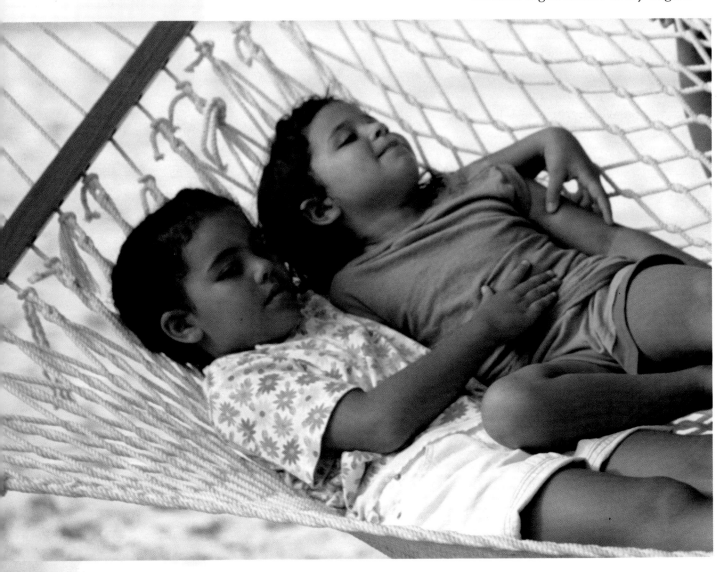

In later life, the need for sleep gradually decreases. People over 70 years of age typically sleep for only about six hours a night and for many, sleep becomes lighter and is prone to frequent disruptions.

All of the above are only broad generalisations – your own or other people's sleeping habits could differ widely from the pattern given. The only important thing to bear in mind is whether or not you are getting the right amount of sleep for you. There is an idea that people who don't need much sleep are somehow more productive than those who sleep for longer periods but this is not necessarily the case. The UK Prime Minister Margaret Thatcher famously claimed to need only four hours of sleep a night, but Albert Einstein by contrast was said to regularly sleep for ten or more hours every night!

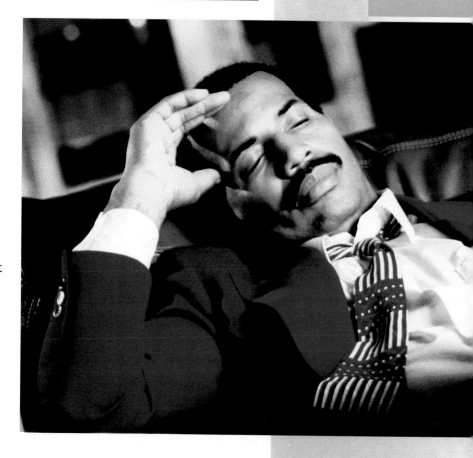

Research into sleep deprivation suggests that the body has inbuilt mechanisms which prevent us from sleeping too much. In experiments where subjects were deprived of sleep for as long as several days, none of the subjects slept for more than 15 hours continuously when they were eventually allowed to sleep. It seems that we can make up for lost sleep time very quickly.

Studies also suggest that very irregular sleep patterns can result in the same irritability and poor concentration associated with a lack of sleep.

Above: there is an idea that people who don't need much sleep are somehow more productive than those who sleep for longer periods but this is not necessarily the case.

WHAT IS INSOMNIA?

Far left: an afternoon nap can sharpen the attention span.

Below: insomnia can include difficulty falling asleep during the night.

A look at a standard dictionary will tell us that the word insomnia derives from the Latin word *insomnis* meaning the prolonged and usually abnormal inability to obtain adequate sleep. Aspects of insomnia can include difficulty falling asleep; waking up frequently during the night with difficulty falling back to sleep; waking up too early in the morning; and waking up feeling unrefreshed by sleep.

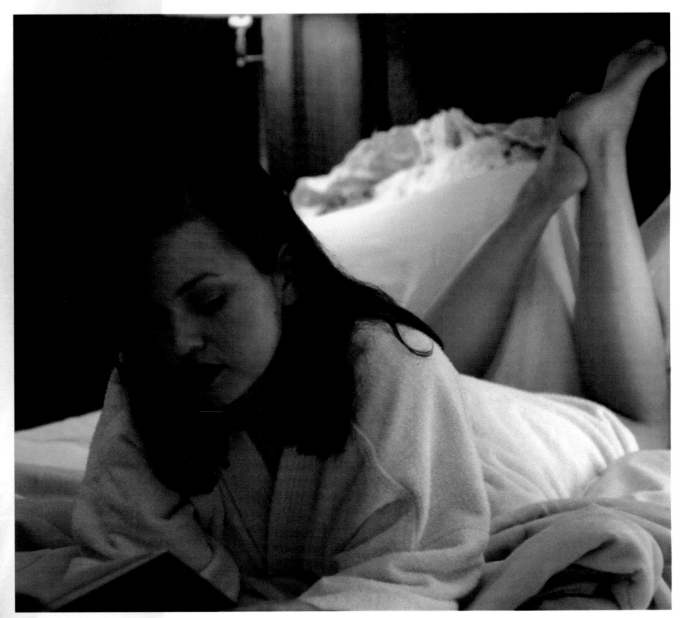

It is important to remember that one or two nights of disrupted sleep does not constitute a problem in itself. The neighbours may have thrown a late-night party or you may be nervous about an imminent driving test and therefore don't get as much sleep as you would like – these are very temporary situations that soon pass. When comparing your own sleep needs with those of other people, many factors should be taken into account. People are very different and each individual's sleeping needs will vary widely. Some people need much more sleep than others.

There are various cultural differences to be considered, too. Some cultures, for instance, traditionally take an afternoon nap or siesta while others do not. Research suggests that an afternoon nap can sharpen the attention span and should not interfere with the night-time sleeping pattern provided the nap is not longer than half an hour. If a longer nap is taken, the body tends to go into a deeper level of sleep which means you are likely to wake up feeling groggy and more tired than before. Older people may also find they nap periodically throughout the day. This is normal but also reduces the amount of time spent sleeping at night.

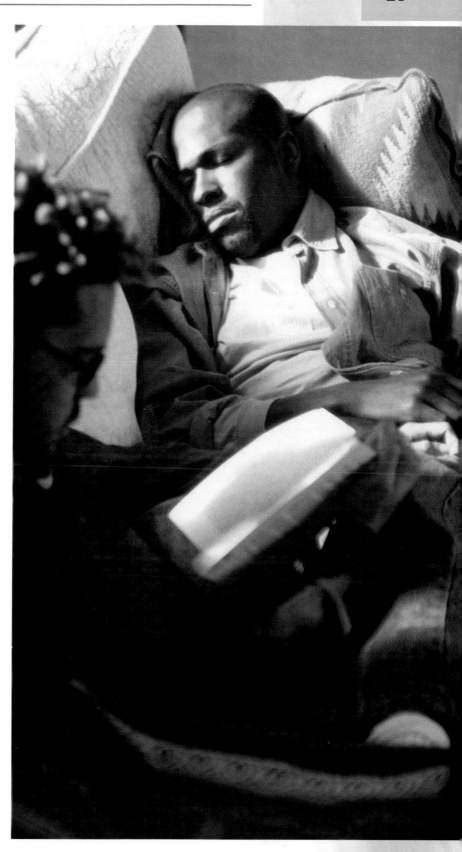

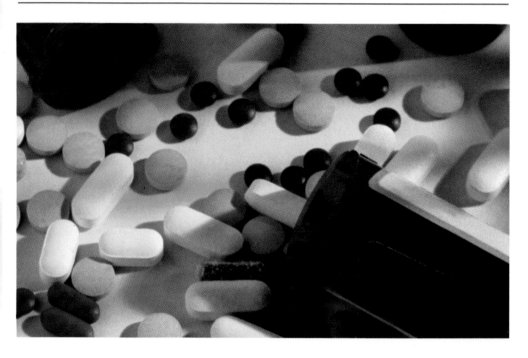

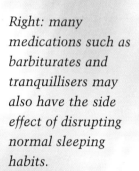

Right: many medications such as barbiturates and tranquillisers may also have the side effect of disrupting normal sleeping habits.

Insomnia comes in many different degrees of severity and can have many causes, but the medical profession generally groups the causes into four main categories:

ENVIRONMENTAL INSOMNIA

This is disruption caused to the sleeping pattern created by external factors in the vicinity or situation around you. These environmental factors may range from noise from a local night club to an uncomfortable bed! Many medications such as barbiturates and tranquillisers may also have the side effect of disrupting normal sleeping habits. (Do not make any changes to prescribed medications without discussing it with your doctor first).

INSOMNIA CAUSED BY A PHYSICAL DISEASES OR PROBLEM

There are a great many physical ailments that can contribute to insomnia. Being in pain in itself will obviously disrupt sleep patterns. Conditions that are also known to produce sleep problems include heart problems, asthma, a prolonged cough, the menopause, a hyperactive thyroid, prostate problems and drug dependency.

INSOMNIA TRIGGERED BY MENTAL ILLNESSES

Mental illness is a common cause of disruption to the sleep pattern. Treatment here must focus primarily on treating the mental disease that is the cause of the problem rather than the insomnia which is just the symptom.

PRIMARY INSOMNIA

Primary insomnia is the medical term for insomnia that has no apparent cause and is actually the main category that most people's sleep problems will fall into. Of course, the other causes of insomnia such as physical pain and environmental factors all have to be eliminated first before placing any sufferer in this particular category. This highlights the need for anyone suffering sleep difficulties to get sound medical advice and to carefully examine their home circumstances before making any assumptions.

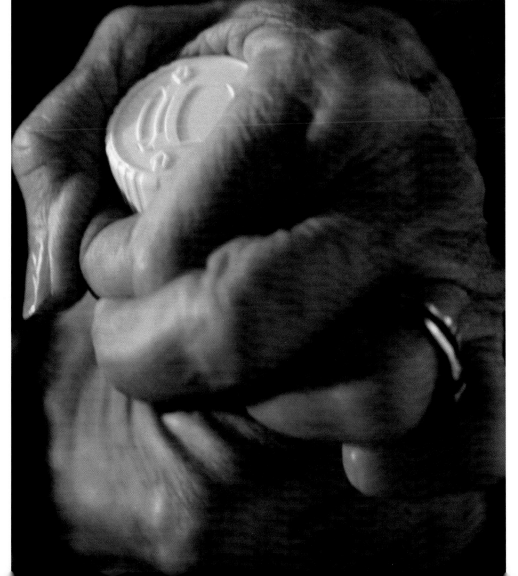

Left: conditions that are also known to produce sleep problems include heart problems, asthma, a prolonged cough, the menopause, a hyperactive thyroid, prostate problems and drug dependency.

All of these categories are merely generalisations and someone suffering from insomnia may well fall into more than one category. For instance, someone who is in physical pain may also feel depressed which exacerbates the sleep situation.

In addition to the causes of insomnia, there are also many levels of the condition to be considered. These tend to be defined in terms of longevity so we have transient insomnia and short-term insomnia right through to chronic insomnia.

Transient insomnia is a temporary condition that all of us are familiar with. One or two nights of disrupted sleep comes under this category. The results will be tiredness and irritability, but the problem is not serious and no treatment is required other than perhaps going to bed earlier than usual the next day or catching up on sleep over a weekend.

Below: someone who is in physical pain may also feel depressed, which exacerbates the sleep situation.

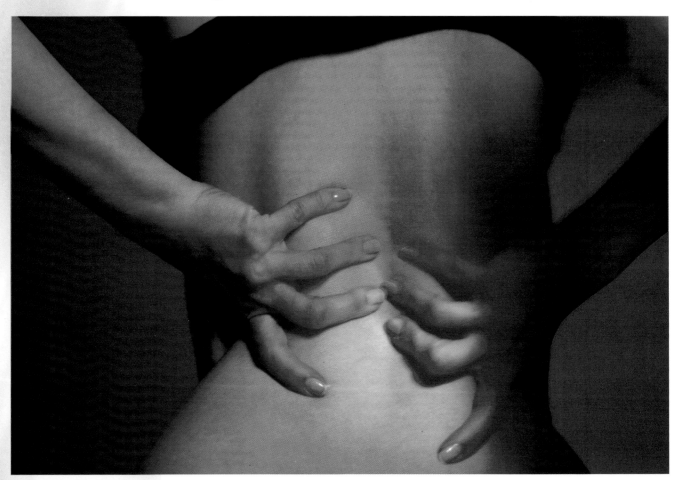

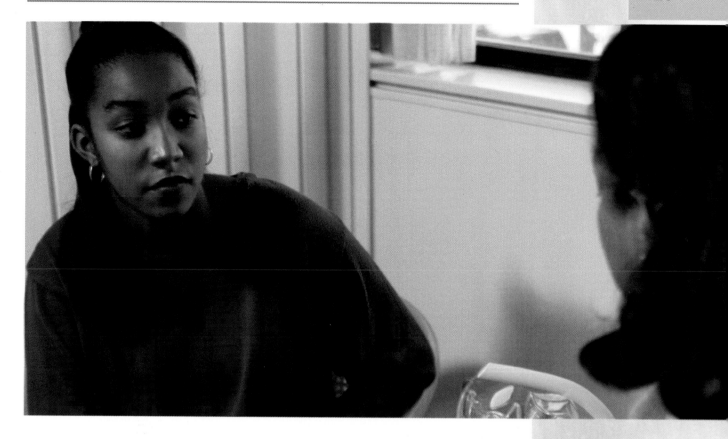

Short-term insomnia is disrupted sleep than can last up to but no longer than three consecutive weeks. This may be caused by the pain of a physical illness or the worry, stress and anxiety caused by some event in our personal lives. Time and an improvement in circumstances may be the only solution possible. But, where there is no improvement after three weeks, the condition may progress into chronic insomnia.

Chronic insomnia occurs when disrupted sleep patterns continue for longer than three continuous weeks. At this level, insomnia becomes a serious enough condition to severely reduce the quality of life of the sufferer. Lack of sleep will inevitably start to affect our general bodily health. Medical treatment is definitely required and the sufferer should contact their doctor without delay to insist on getting a diagnosis. Actually getting an accurate diagnosis may be a lengthy and laborious process in itself because all aspects of the sufferer's lifestyle must be examined in order to track down the cause.

Above: lack of sleep will inevitably start to affect our general bodily health.

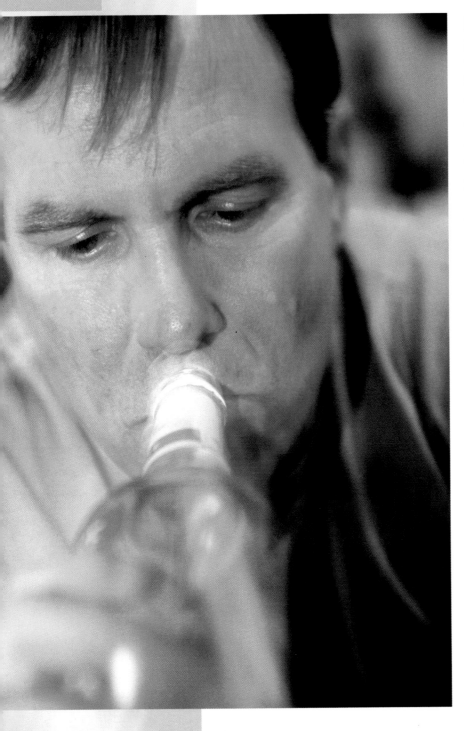

progress of the condition. If possible, this diary should begin when sleep problems first start to be an inconvenience and should then be filled in every day. As soon as you realise you have a sleep problem, take a note of the day this first began as near as possible. Record the daily details of what time you got to bed, when you got up and the length and quality of the sleep experienced that night. Also record what you ate each day, whether or not you smoked tobacco, drank alcohol or coffee and your feelings during the day. Record what is happening in your life. It is important to include details of any medication taken and perhaps how much exercise you took. This will prove invaluable both for yourself and to help any practitioner understand your individual circumstances.

Some famous insomniacs:

Napoleon
Catherine the Great
Winston Churchill
Charles Dickens
Thomas Edison
Cary Grant
Marilyn Monroe
Vincent Van Gogh.

Above: excess alcohol can have an adverse effect on sleep.

Most authorities agree that one important step a sufferer of chronic insomnia should take is to keep a sleep diary to record the

We are all familiar with the effects of losing just one night of restful sleep and the irritability and lack of concentration that results. Sufferers of chronic insomnia who go through extended periods of disrupted sleep can add many more symptoms to this list such as depression and even paranoia. However, there are many other conditions which generally occur at night and either happen during sleep itself or while in the twilight realms somewhere between sleep and wakefulness.

Below: there are many symptoms of disrupted sleep such as depression and even paranoia.

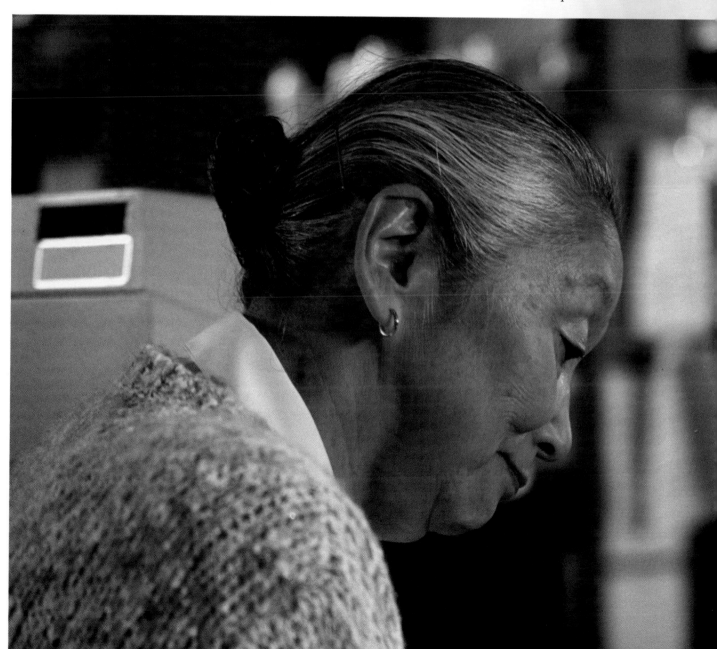

SNORING

Snoring is often considered to be something of a joke except by the unfortunate partner sharing a bed with the snorer – and sometimes even by the neighbours! Snoring can reach levels of up to 80 decibels or so – a level that can be equated with industrial noise pollution! How on earth the snoring person is not woken up by the sound of their own snoring is a mystery that many a long-suffering partner has contemplated during the long hours of darkness. More than a third of adults snore and most of the culprits are men although the number of women who snore increases after the menopause. But it is not just the partner of the snorer who suffers from this affliction. The snorer too may feel tired and inefficient the next day. Snoring is caused by a blockage in either the throat or nose. Once we are asleep, the muscles in the neck and throat become relaxed, allowing the soft palate at the back of the throat to vibrate with each intake of breath. These muscles become weaker with age so the propensity for snoring also increases over time. Having a cold or the flu can produce temporary bouts of snoring as can allergies, polyps and enlarged adenoids and tonsils. Being overweight, smoking and consuming large quantities of alcohol will also increase the likelihood of snoring. Sleeping on your back will not help either.

Below: how on earth the snoring person is not woken up by the sound of their own snoring is a mystery.

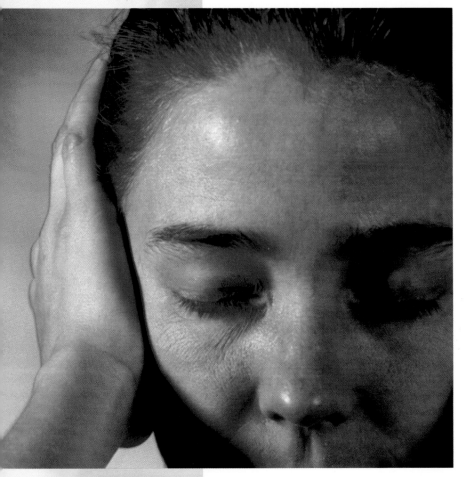

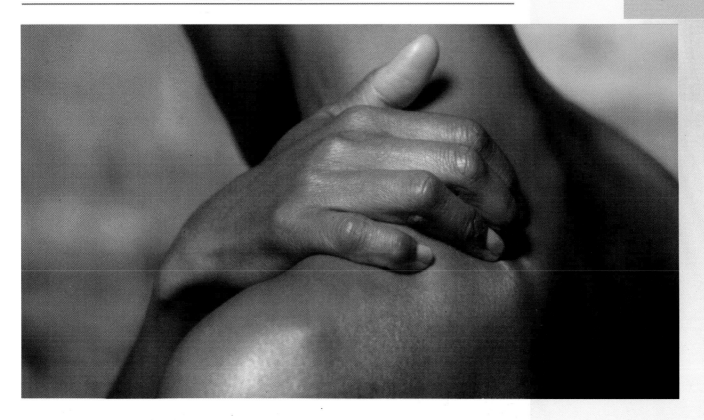

Snoring, although highly annoying, is not generally a health problem. However, the more severe variant called apnea is certainly considered with more alarm. With cases of apnea, the sleeper's breathing passages become temporarily blocked because the soft palate tissues are being sucked closed. This produces loud snoring and frequent bouts of choking and the apnea sufferer may suddenly wake up gasping for breath. Very often the sufferer wakes up so momentarily that they do not even remember it. Each attack can last anything from ten to 90 seconds and may reoccur hundreds of times every night! If these bouts of apnea happen during REM sleep when the body is temporarily almost paralysed, the body takes longer to respond to the lack of air. The sufferer will then wake up in the morning exhausted and often with a headache through lack of oxygen. To be regularly deprived of oxygen is clearly a serious situation, in addition to the dangers of not getting sufficient REM sleep. Apnea sufferers live with an increased chance of having a heart attack or stroke. Fortunately, the most severe cases of apnea are rare.

Above: the apnea sufferer will wake up in the morning exhausted and often with a headache.

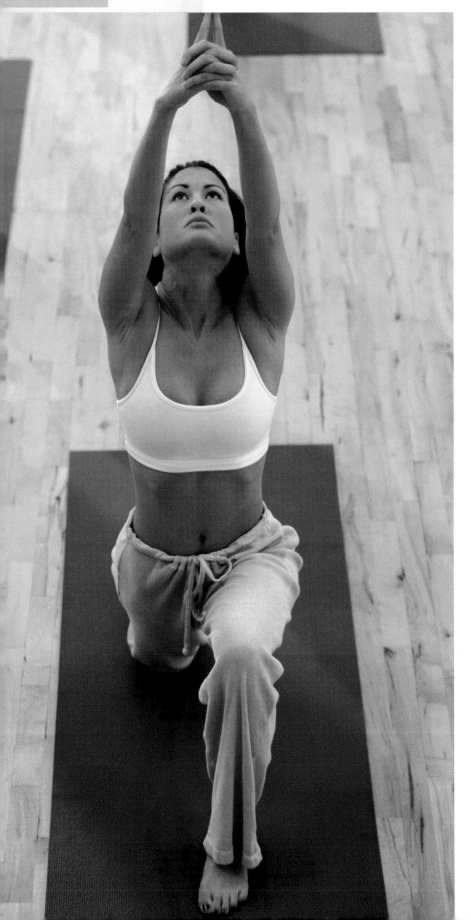

The causes of apnea are similar to those that cause normal snoring. If you suffer from either condition, you should stop smoking and maintain a healthy body weight. There are no particular drug treatments that have proved to be effective in treating apnea, but improving the quality of breathing is an obvious place to start. Most people in everyday life don't breath deeply enough anyway so taking up yoga or meditation, with sensible breathing exercises, could prove very helpful. Nasal dilators used by athletes to improve their oxygen intake may also be effective. These can be either plasters placed across the nose or plastic clips that are attached to the outside of the nose. Sufferers of severe apnea may be encouraged to use a CPAP (continuous positive airway pressure) machine that works by delivering oxygen through a nasal mask. Surgery is another possible, if last resort, treatment.

NIGHTMARES

As we discussed earlier, even though we are all familiar with and have experience of the dream state, the subject of dreams is one where, despite thousands of years of exploration and research, we still have more questions than answers. It is thought that we all dream every night although some people remember their dreams more often and more vividly than others. Some people can regale others with tales of their epic adventures almost every night whereas some insist they never dream at all. Some even have the same recurring dream year after year. The one type of dream we are all guaranteed to remember, though, and which we have all experienced, is the bad dream – the nightmare.

It seems that all of us have had nightmares at one time or another and a few unfortunate individuals are plagued regularly with night terrors. Children are more prone to having nightmares than any other group, but for a substantial amount of people their nightmares continue into adulthood.

Far left: yoga or meditation, with sensible breathing exercises, could prove helpful.

Below: the one type of dream we are all guaranteed to remember, and which we have all experienced, is the bad dream – the nightmare.

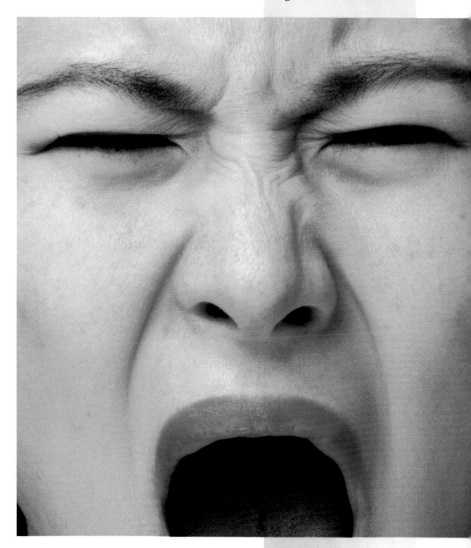

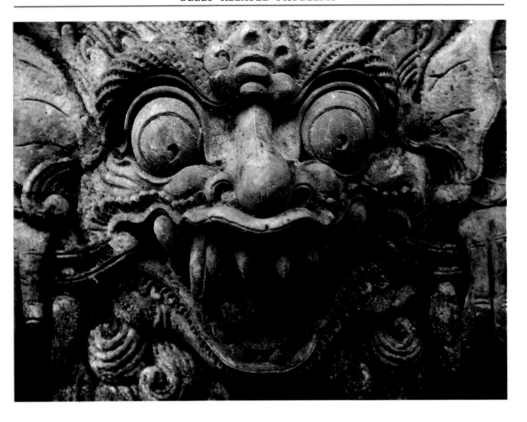

Above: nightmares are thought of by some as visitations by evil spirits and demons.

Far right: nightmares can be a symptom of repressed fear, guilt or grief.

Virtually all dreams can be judged to be somewhat strange by the standards of our everyday waking life but, whatever the subject matter, the hallmark of a nightmare is that the dreamer feels a very real and profound sense of threat and fear. Sleepers in the grip of a nightmare often find themselves in increasingly disturbing circumstances from which there seems no escape until, at the climax of the horror, they are jolted into sudden wakefulness often sitting bolt upright in bed feeling either hot and sweaty or in a cold sweat.

Many ancient cultures that regarded the dream state as a time to commune with the gods and spirits naturally thought of nightmares as visitations by evil spirits and demons. The popular view in modern western countries is that nightmares are a symptom of repressed fear, guilt or grief that bubbles to the surface when the conscious mind is unable to create any distractions from the pain. It is certainly true that people can experience nightmares after going through a particularly traumatic event such as bereavement or after a bad accident. Drugs, alcohol or even eating shortly before bedtime can also trigger nightmares.

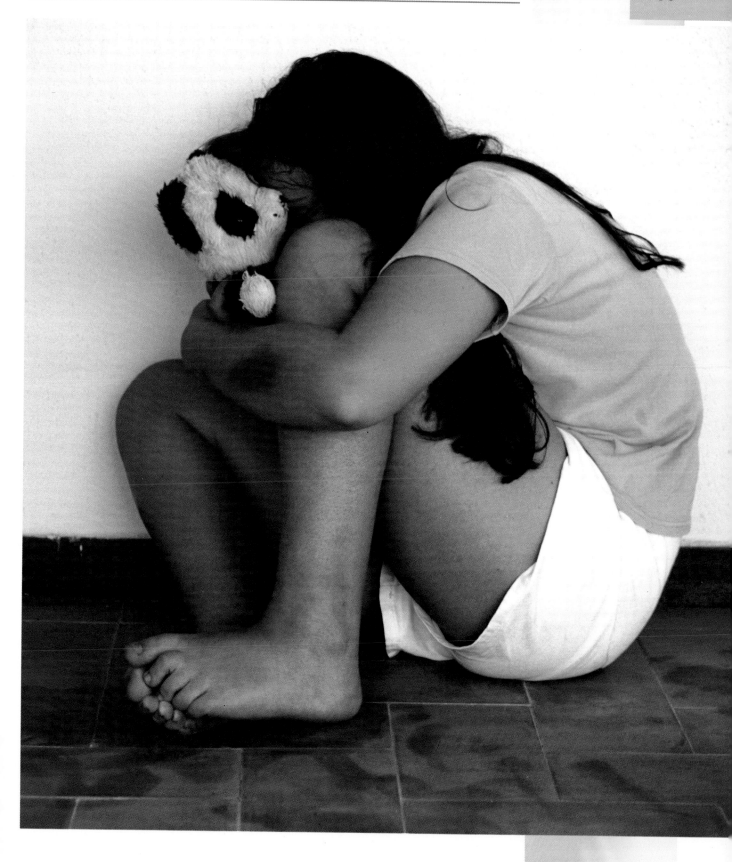

Right: dreaming you are being chased symbolises something you are running away from.

Far right: dreamng you are naked can signify a lack of confidence.

Many psychologists now believe nightmares are one way the subconscious mind can alert us to issues that need to be resolved in our lives. For this reason it is better to face up to our nightmares even though it is tempting to try to forget them. Bookshops are now groaning under the weight of books claiming to decipher our dreams. These are based on comparisons of many people's dream imagery. These dream interpretation books may have some merit provided they are used as food for thought and not seen as a definitive guide to the subconscious. Each person has their own language of dream imagery based on their own personal and emotional experiences so what is a negative symbol for one person may be a positive one for someone else. The language of our dreams is best understood once we understand it is our emotions that are being dramatised. Even so, there are some common themes in nightmares that are worth mentioning here.

Falling from a height or through the air:

This may be an expression of repressed feelings of inferiority, insecurity or instability.

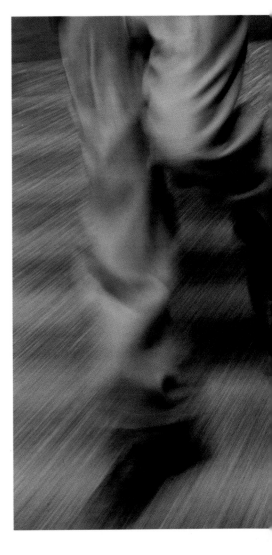

Being chased:
Whatever is chasing you is a symbol of something you are running away from in your waking life. We are always dealing with aspects of ourselves. This would signify the need to face up to whatever is frightening you – maybe it's not really that scary after all.

Discovering that you are naked or half-dressed in a public place:
This is a very basic expression of feelings of self-consciousness – we are being exposed to the prying eyes of others. This would signify a lack of confidence with regard to some aspect of your social interaction with others.

Taking an exam for which you don't know the answers:
This denotes feeling unprepared for the tests of life. This can be due to feeling inadequate or feeling judged by others.

Teeth falling out:
From the time as infants when we are teething and get our milk teeth to the time of our old age when our teeth fall out, teeth symbolise changes in the stages of our life. How we feel about these changes will be reflected in the dream. Are we traumatised, or relieved? Are teeth knocked out or lost or cause pain? These dreams can often signify feelings of powerlessness or impotence.

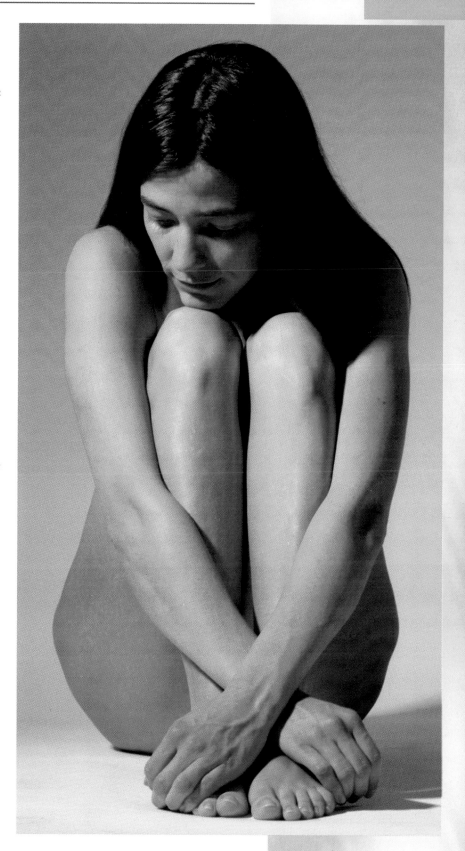

Remember that the above are only suggestions and the occurrence of these images in your nightmares may well have entirely different meanings for you. If you suffer from nightmares and want to get to the bottom of them, one suggestion is to sleep with a pen and paper by the bed and write down what you remember of your dreams each morning whether your dreams are nightmares or not. In time, your own private dream language will become clear as you reflect on how your dream time and waking time interact. With practice you can also learn to consciously recognise when you are dreaming without waking up. This is known as lucid dreaming. In this lucid dreaming state you can learn to explore and eventually control the dream from the inside as it were. If nightmares become a severe problem, you should see a doctor or psychologist, as you may need an objective opinion.

Below: write down what you remember of your dreams each morning.

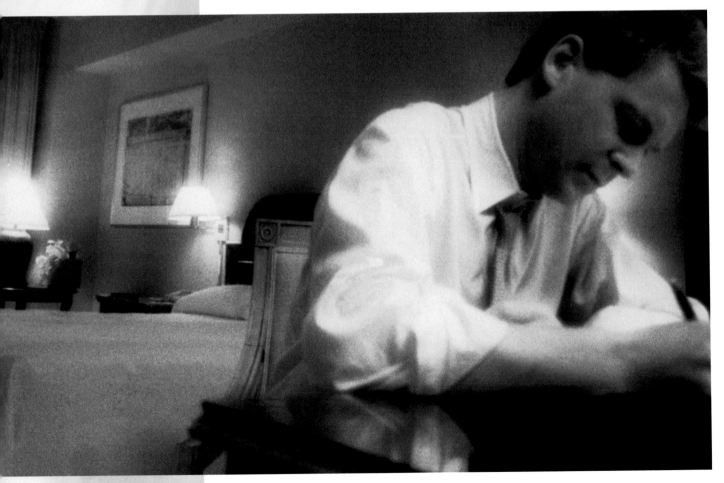

SLEEPWALKING

Sleepwalking or somnambulism is a well-known condition where the still-sleeping person gets up and walks about. These episodes of sleepwalking can last for anything up to about an hour (usually during the first half of the night) during which the sufferer – still in deep sleep – can perform quite complicated and protracted tasks. It is not unknown for the sleepwalker to get up, get dressed, go out of the house and even drive a car considerable distances before waking up! Children are more likely than adults to suffer from this strange condition, and more boys than girls are afflicted. About 15 per cent of people sleepwalk at some time in their lives. There is also evidence to suggest that sleepwalking has a hereditary factor. Most children who sleepwalk grow out of the condition naturally, but those who continue into adulthood are more likely to suffer from stress and anxiety. People who sleep erratically such as shift workers and those who go through extended periods of sleeplessness are more prone to sleepwalk. There is little that can be done to prevent sleepwalking other than to relieve any stress that may be an aggravating or contributing factor and to avoid activities that may confuse the body's internal clock such as drinking alcohol. The accepted wisdom now is that it is best not to wake the sleepwalker up if possible, but rather to guide them gently back to bed while giving reassurance that all is well. Removing potentially dangerous items from the bedroom and locking the door may also be prudent to limit any extremes of activity.

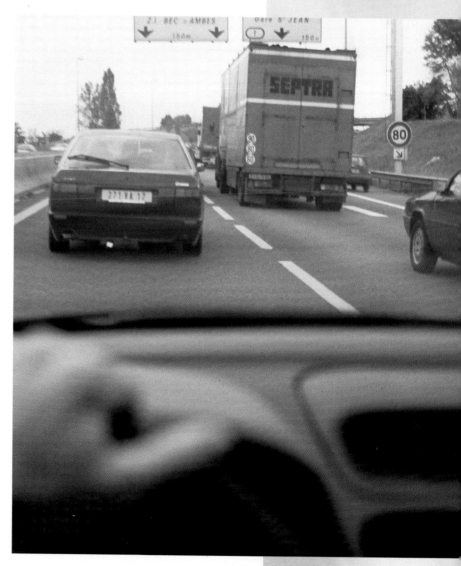

Below: the sleepwalker may get up, get dressed, go out of the house and even drive a car.

BEDWETTING

Far right: Narcolepsy is a very rare condition where the victim can suddenly fall asleep at any time.

Below: stress is the major cause of bedwetting and can become a vicious circle if the parents react by punishing the child.

Like sleepwalking, bedwetting or enuresis tends to run in families. It is more common in boys than in girls and it usually ceases to be a problem once children are into their adolescence. The older a child is, the more distressed they are by the problem. There is rarely a physical cause of the bed-wetting and if there is, there will be other daytime symptoms that alert the parents to the problem. Stress is the major cause of bed-wetting and can become a vicious circle if the parents react by punishing the child. Events such as trouble at school or changing schools, stress at home such as arguing siblings or parents could all be triggers for the condition. Usually, love and patient understanding is all that is required to gradually remedy the situation. If an older child who has no history of bed-wetting suddenly develops the problem, it may be wise to get some medical advice as it may be evidence of a urinary-tract infection. Encourage any child who wets the bed not to drink before bedtime but don't stop them drinking if they are thirsty. There are experts in the USA who have had success in teaching bladder control to severe sufferers and some have had success with the drug imipramine, an antidepressant that has the side effect of improving bladder control. Some parents have had results using a pad and buzzer device in the child's bed. This teaches the child to associate going to the toilet with waking up.

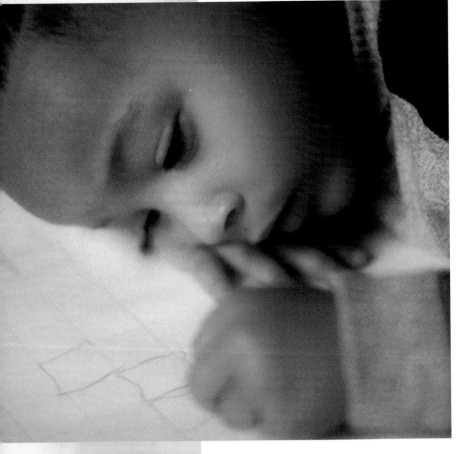

NARCOLEPSY

Narcolepsy is a very rare condition where the victim can suddenly fall asleep at any time without having any control over the situation at all. This can happen even while driving a car or while having sex – situations where adrenalin in the bloodstream would be expected to keep people awake. The sufferer may lose all strength in their muscles immediately before an attack and then have instant paralysis similar to that experienced in REM sleep. Less than one per cent of the population suffer from this inconvenient condition – one famous sufferer being the actress Natasha Kinski. The dangers of suddenly falling asleep are obvious and doctors may prescribe amphetamines to increase alertness. Unfortunately, narcolepsy is incurable and is largely genetically determined. Strong emotions may bring on an attack and the condition is at its worst in the years immediately after adolescence.

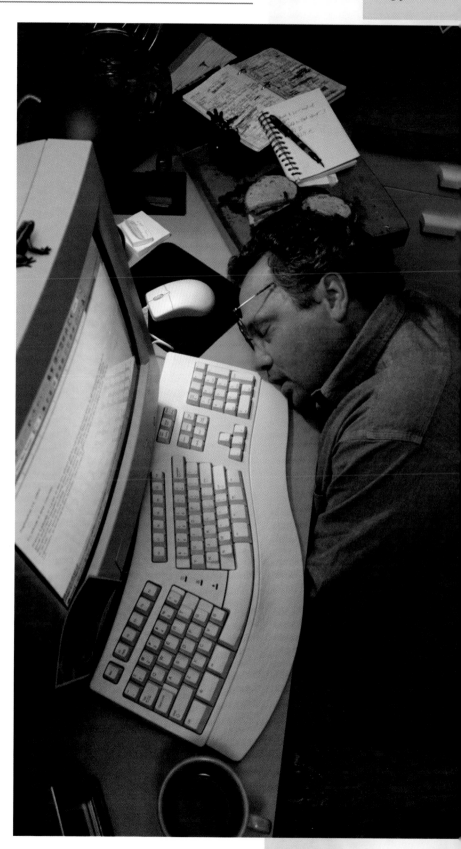

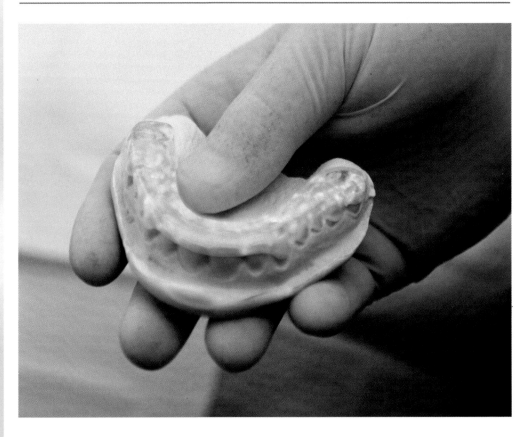

Right: teeth grinding and clenching can often be remedied by regularly wearing a shield in the mouth overnight which the dentist can provide.

TEETH GRINDING

Teeth grinding or bruxism is much more common than is usually thought. In fact it is estimated that 80 to 90 per cent of adults and children go through periods of either teeth grinding or clenching the teeth during sleep. Most people who grind or clench their teeth do not know they are doing it since the practice does not necessarily wake the grinder up. The sufferer may wake up in the morning with a headache or feeling unrested. It is often the partner of the teeth grinder who first notices the problem since the noise can be quite loud. The majority of people who suffer from this condition are alerted to it by a dentist since both teeth grinding and clenching can damage the teeth. If the condition continues unchecked for too long, damage to both the teeth and jaw alignment can create long-term problems that can throw the whole body out of balance. The condition is often linked to stress and anxiety, but this has not been proved. Teeth grinding and clenching can often be remedied by regularly wearing a shield in the mouth overnight which the dentist can provide.

RESTLESS LEG SYNDROME

Restless leg syndrome is an essentially harmless but very common problem where the sufferer feels an irritating agitation in the legs while lying in bed. This can feel like something between an ache and a tingle in the legs that just won't go away. The sufferer can't lie still and may feel a need to get up and walk around for a while to relieve the restlessness. If this becomes too regular, it can become disruptive both for sufferers and these who share a bed with them. The actual causes of restless leg syndrome are unknown, but reducing alcohol and caffeine intake and taking more exercise may help. The problem may also be aggravated by diabetes, anaemia or renal failure. These are conditions that clearly do need medical treatment even though the restless leg syndrome itself does not. Many people find that massaging the legs for half an hour or so before bedtime provides relief from restless leg syndrome although this is not always the case.

It is estimated that around 80 per cent of restless leg syndrome sufferers are also victims of periodic limb movement syndrome (PLMS). Here the legs and sometimes the arms twitch every 30 seconds or so. Some people can suffer from PLMS without being afflicted with restless leg syndrome. Again, PLMS is not a serious condition and the sufferer is not usually woken up by the twitching. However, the partner of the PLMS sufferer will naturally be disturbed, while the sufferer's muscles are not getting the rest that sleep should bring. As with restless leg syndrome, the causes of PLMS are unknown although good exercise patterns (well before bedtime) and reducing tea and coffee intake should help. Taking calcium and iron supplements may help, too.

Below: reducing tea and coffee intake should help restless leg syndrome.

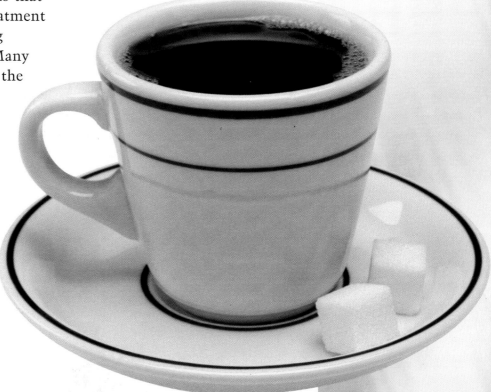

CRAMPS

Yet another limb condition to afflict some sleepers is leg or foot cramps during the night. These may be caused by poor circulation and or lack of exercise. There are various medical conditions that may produce cramps so it is best to see a doctor if cramps are a regular problem. Some sufferers find that evening primrose oil provides some relief as does homeopathic cuprum. Vitamin E helps the circulation so consider taking this as a supplement or eating more avocados and nuts as they are high in vitamin E.

Right: another limb condition to afflict some sleepers is leg or foot cramps.

Far right: we now live in a high speed and global age where international commerce and electronic communications dictate that life should go on 24 hours a day.

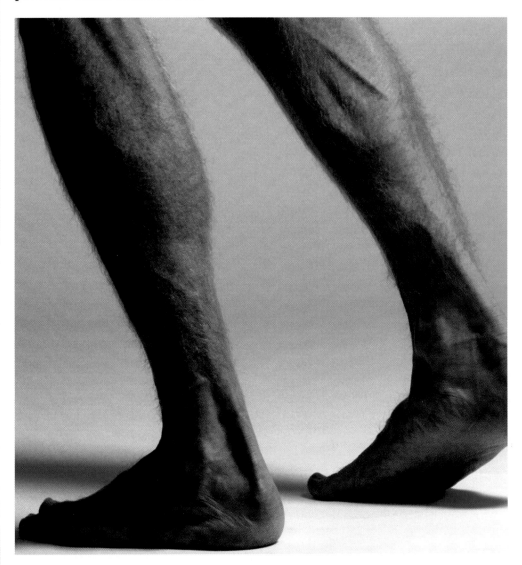

YOUR SLEEPING ENVIRONMENT

One of the biggest enemies of healthy, natural sleep has been the invention of electric lighting. Before this, people tended to go to sleep when it got dark and got up with the sun each morning since even gas lighting was dangerous and fiddly. Now we live in a high speed and global age where international commerce and electronic communications dictate that life should go on 24 hours a day. High-speed air travel can take us through many time zones in a matter of hours. The fast pace of life is used as a synonym for youth and success – if you can't keep up, you're past it! If you get tired, take a drug to keep you awake. If you can't stand the noise, you're too old. Whereas once people waited patiently for the post to arrive, now if an email is not replied to within a couple of hours, people think they are being ignored. Given this chaotic and unnatural environment, it is perhaps not surprising that so many people feel cut off from the rhythms of nature.

All this highlights the need to create a safe and comfortable sanctuary for yourself where you can relax, unwind and ultimately, sleep.

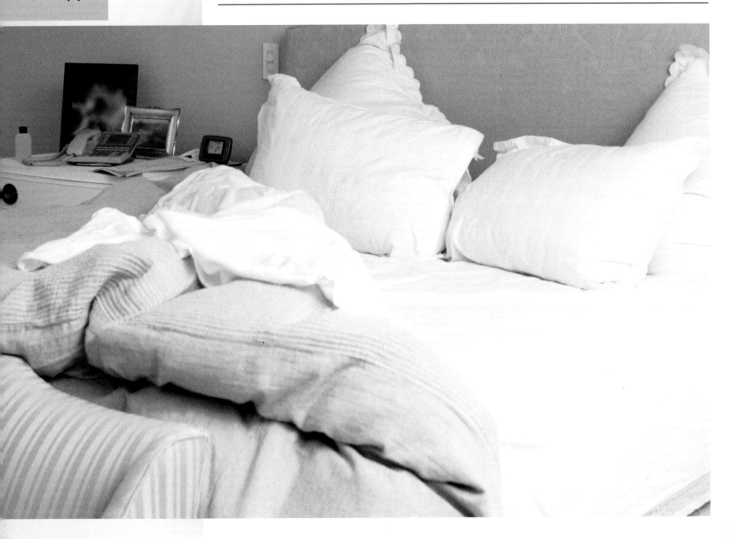

Above: think carefully about the type of bed that suits you best.

BEDS AND BEDDING

Since you will spend a third of your life lying in one, you need to think carefully about the type of bed that suits you best. There are, of course, many different kinds of sleeping surfaces and coverings used around the world dependent on weather and cultural tradition. In the western world, the traditional bed base and mattress dominates the market. The recommended life span of the average bed is ten years, but few of us heed that advice. Most people keep their bed for around double this time even though most mattresses will have deteriorated by about 75 per cent after ten years. If you wake up in the morning unrested and plagued by aches and pains, it may be time to consider investing in a new bed.

When you go to the shop, do not allow yourself to be rushed by sales staff. Beds and mattresses can be expensive so you need not feel guilty about taking your time. The first thing to consider when buying a new bed is the size. A bed should be as wide as possible even if you sleep alone. Preferably, a bed needs to be about six inches longer than its tallest occupant. The type of base for the bed depends on the degree of firmness you prefer. These can range from springs similar to those used in the mattress itself, through to hard wooden slats or metal bars. More important, though, is the type of mattress you choose. The general rule is not too hard or too soft. A good bed will allow your spine to settle into its natural S shape. Test a mattress by lying on it on your back and then slide your hand under the small of your back. If the mattress is too hard, your hand will move around freely. If the mattress is too soft, you will not be able to slide your hand in at all. If the mattress is just right, your hand will slide in and fit comfortably. Most mattresses have many springs inside and the more springs that are independently sprung, the better the support will usually be. Alternative fillings can include polyurethane foam or latex. One important thing is that the mattress must be able to drain away the pint or so of water each of us loses every night. A mattress covering made of natural fibres will cope with moisture well. When you think you have settled on your choice, lie on the bed in the shop for about ten minutes to see if you still feel comfortable before parting with your money. Once in use at home, your mattress should be turned over every few months to keep it in good order.

Below: lie on the bed in the shop for about ten minutes to see if you still feel comfortable.

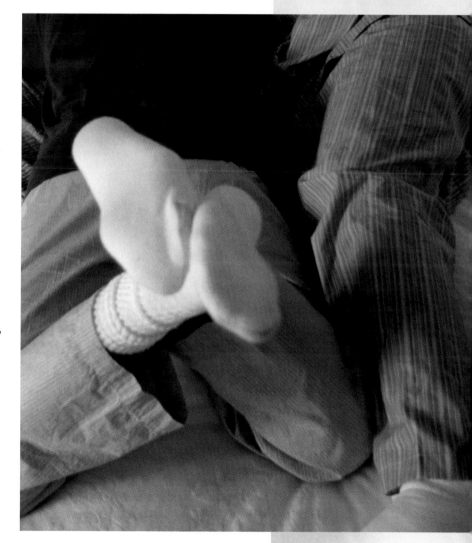

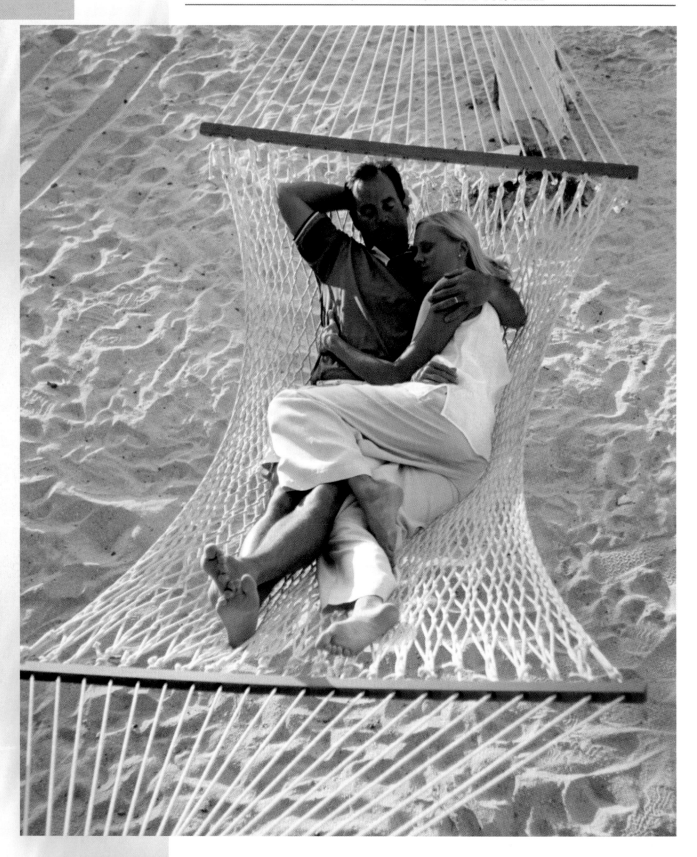

As an alternative to the traditional western bed base, you could consider a Japanese-style futon. These are made of layers of cotton wadding covered with calico and laid on a base made of wooden slats. This type of bed provides good support and can often convert into a useful sofa. The cotton mattress does require a good shake every so often to avoid the cotton layers forming into solid lumps.

Water beds are made of vinyl and are filled with water. The benefit of water beds is that they provide great support since they distribute weight evenly. They are also hygienic and non-allergic.

Hammocks are perhaps a less common alternative to the traditional bed. The benefits are the soothing rocking motion they provide and a good circulation of air. They can be easily packed away, but hammocks do need a large room to accommodate each end.

Once you have decided on the type of bed you want, you can think about the kind of pillows and bedding to go with it.

There are many kinds of pillows to choose from depending on your preferred sleeping position. The idea is to keep your head at the same angle to your shoulders that you have standing up. In general, if you sleep on your back, a medium pillow is best. If you sleep on your side, you need a firmer pillow. If you normally sleep on your stomach, a softer pillow is less of a strain on your neck. Feather pillows mould better to the shape of your head, but these don't last so long as synthetic fibres and can produce allergic reactions in some people.

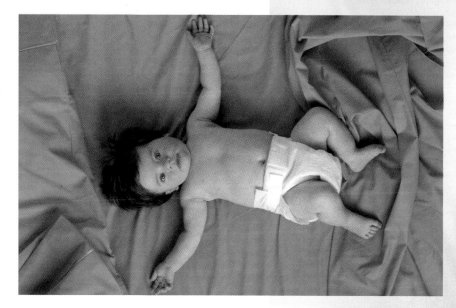

Pillows made from synthetic fibres or foam will not aggravate allergies and are washable. Some people like to put a small pillow filled with herbs or hops inside the main pillow to promote good sleep. Babies should not be given pillows until they are over one year old to avoid any danger of suffocation.

Above: babies should not be given pillows until they are over one year old to avoid any danger of suffocation.

Far left: hammocks are perhaps a less common alternative to the traditional bed.

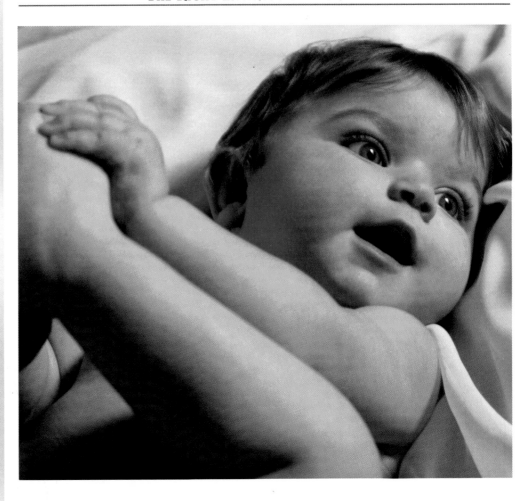

Right: cotton sheets and blankets should be used for babies.

Your next choice is the type of bedding. Most people in the western world now prefer duvets because it is easier to make the bed. Like pillows, duvets can be either synthetic or filled with feathers. Natural fibres allow the skin to breathe better, but will wear out faster than synthetic fibres and will cause an allergic reaction in some people. Many people prefer blankets and sheets as these can be added or taken off to suit the weather. Again, natural fibres allow the skin to breath properly. Cotton sheets and blankets should be used for babies. If you need extra heat in the bed, get a good quality hot water bottle or a hot lover. Electric blankets emit electro-magnetic radiation that is detrimental to health and are best avoided.

Once you are sorted out with bed and bedding, it's time to take a look at the wider environment starting with the bedroom itself.

BEDROOM DESIGN

How comfortable and conducive to sleep is your bedroom environment? The bedroom should be a peaceful sanctuary used for sleep and sex only. In this space you should be able to be completely alone to relax or to explore private intimacy with your lover. The bedroom should not double up as an office, study or general storage area. However, we do not live in an ideal world, and many people will have to compromise somewhat. Even so, you should maintain the idea of a sacred space and clear away everything inappropriate at night.

Given a house with some flexibility, the first thing to consider is which room to make the bedroom. Clearly, a room furthest away from the noise of roads and street lighting may be the best choice. You should also consider which direction the windows face. A south- or north-facing bedroom window will get steady light all day, but the bedroom is unlikely to be occupied during most of the day. A west-facing window will capture the sunset. The most natural placement for a bedroom window is east-facing. This will capture the energising sunrise and will therefore encourage a natural waking rhythm that is in tune with the elements.

Below: the bedroom should be a peaceful sanctuary used for sleep and sex only.

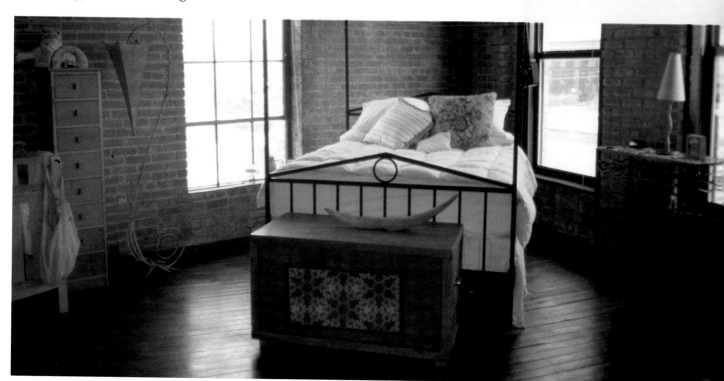

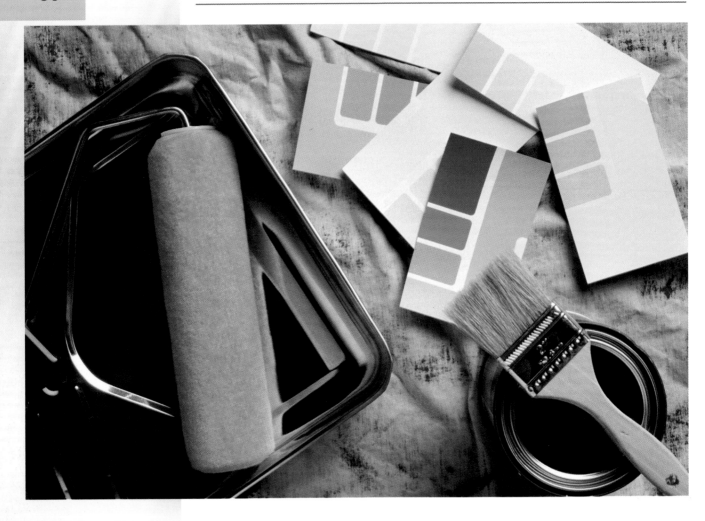

Above: you need to consider the colour of the bedroom.

The next thing you need to consider is the colour of the bedroom. Colour has an enormously powerful effect on our mood, so choosing the right colour for you is very important. You should bear in mind that the bedroom is usually intended for the dual purposes of sleep and sex, which are very different moods! A balance between these two functions must therefore be struck. Clearly, we all have different tastes and you must select colours you like, but there are general rules to colour that are worth bearing in mind.

Some people are afraid to make colour choices in case they change their mind later and therefore plump for white walls and ceiling. This is OK provided a fair amount of colour is introduced elsewhere in curtains, carpet, bedding and pictures etc. But, an over white bedroom is somewhat stark and sterile and is not the most sensual of environments – so be adventurous!

Blue – Blue is a warning colour used for the lights of emergency vehicles the world over. It is not restful and is not conducive to sleep.

Green – Light greens are restful and are often used in prisons and hospitals to calm people down. Darker greens can be oppressive though.

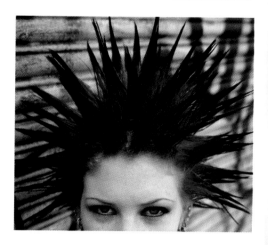

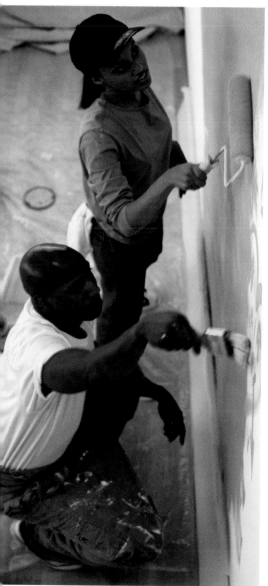

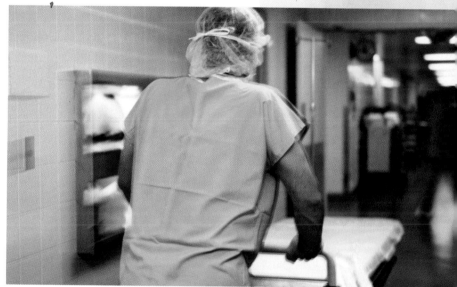

Red – Reds are very stimulating colours and have strong associations with sex. This may cater for one function of the bedroom, but will not promote restful sleep.

Above: light green is restful and calms people down.

Purple – Purple is perhaps a little harsh for the bedroom, but softer lilacs and mauves can be very restful and would be good choices.

Below: bright yellow is very active.

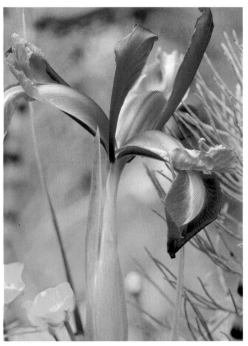

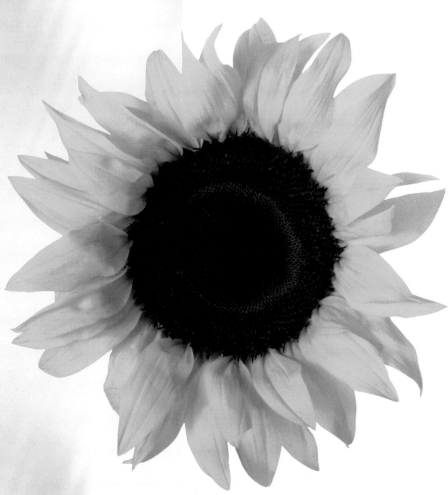

Yellow – Bright yellow is very active and may be more suitable for kitchens than bedrooms. Pale yellows and oranges may be restful.

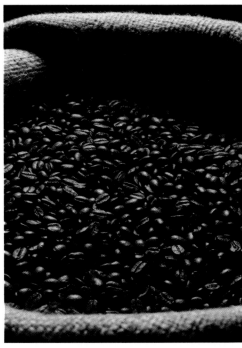

Brown – Dark browns may be rather muddy, but beiges are restful and are popular bedroom choices.

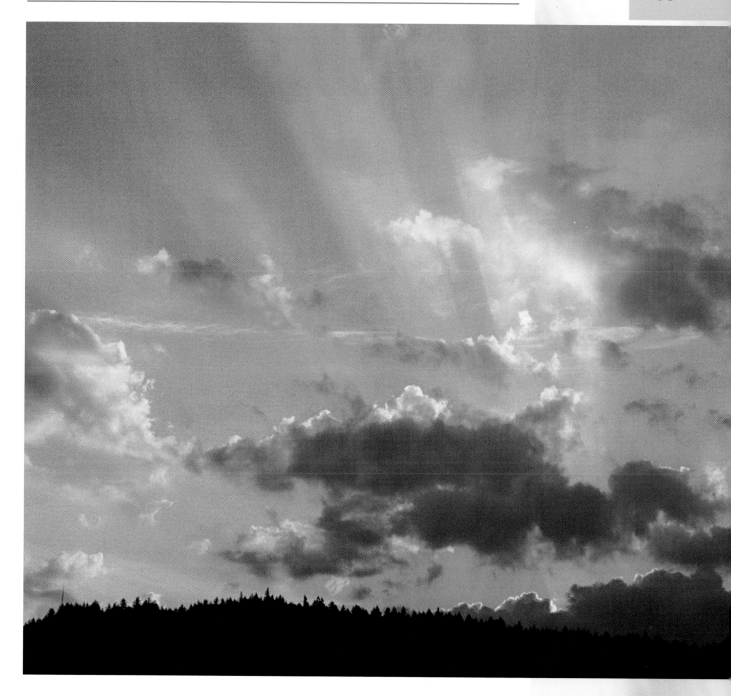

Pink – Warm pinks and peach colours are perhaps ideal bedroom colours as they are restful and also contain enough red to cater for any sensual function of the bedroom.

In general, bright colours are not recommended for promoting sleep whereas softer colours, pastels and creams work well.

Above: warm pinks and peach colours are restful.

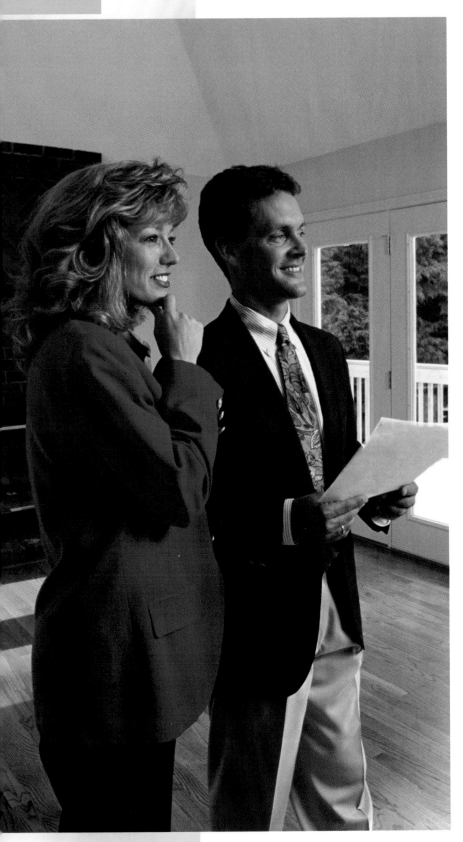

Your next consideration is what to put in your bedroom other than the bed itself – or rather, what should be left out of your bedroom, since clutter is the enemy of peaceful sleep. One approach that may be useful here is the ancient Chinese art of Feng Shui.

Feng Shui (pronounced "fung shway") is a traditional art and science that is based on the understanding that health, wealth and prosperity can be increased by harmonising with the universal streams of energy that flow through everything that exists. Modern man-made structures are usually built with little understanding of these principals and often create disrupted energy fields that alienate people from the abundance that is offered by the universe. Feng Shui, used for thousands of years in the East, has recently become increasingly popular in the West both for homes and offices. Feng Shui is a complex science and the best way of using it is to employ a Feng Shui practitioner to come to your house. However, there are basic things you can do yourself. The section below gives general advice on bedroom design drawing on Feng Shui principles.

For instance, make sure your bedroom is free of clutter so that the energy can flow freely. All clothes and toiletries should be stored out of sight and remove everything that is not relevant to bedroom activities such as computers. It is probably unrealistic to eliminate all electrical devices from the bedroom, but try to keep these to a minimum since they all emit electromagnetic radiation that is detrimental to your health. If possible, replace all mains-powered devices with battery-operated ones. If you live in a single room or studio flat, use a screen or curtain to partition off the sleeping area. Don't have mirrors facing the bed or, better still, place mirrors inside a wardrobe unless your room is an uneven shape. In this case place the mirror where there is a corner missing. Since energy flows between windows and doors, don't place your bed in between these areas. If possible, have the bed where you can see the door, but not directly in front of it. In a small room this may not be possible, so hang a wind chime between the door and the bed to create a symbolic energy break. Also, make sure your bed has space underneath to allow energy to flow between the bed and the floor. Avoid placing pictures and bookshelves above the head of the bed and don't have the bed against or under a window.

Lighting is a much-neglected but important way of changing the dynamics of any space. Firstly, try to place the bed so that the sun does not shine directly on the bed itself. When it comes to choosing lights, go for bedside lamps and up-lighters rather than an overhead central bulb. Windows should have heavy curtains preferably lined with white fabric to reflect back the sunlight when needed. Double glazing is an effective way of shutting out unwanted noise.

Far left: Feng Shui has become increasingly popular in the west both for homes and offices.

Below: go for bedside lamps and up-lighters rather than an overhead central bulb.

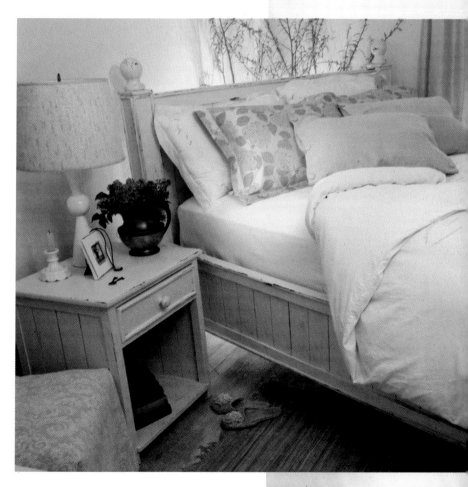

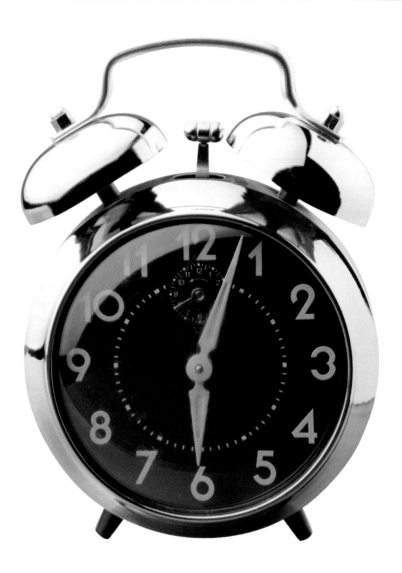

Right: we all know the feeling of resignation when the alarm clock signals it is time to get up.

Anyone living near to a busy road or night club will be painfully aware of the extent to which unwanted noise has an adverse effect on sleeping patterns. It is clear to all of us that a reasonably quiet environment provides fewer distractions and makes it easier to drop off to sleep. We also all know the irritation caused by sudden nocturnal sounds that wake us up – and the feeling of resignation when the alarm clock signals that it is time to get up for work. It would be wrong, however, to assume that complete silence is the ideal to aspire to. For one thing, few of us live in areas where this is a realistic expectation. Also many people find total silence and darkness rather disconcerting and this may actually keep us awake. Each individual reacts differently.

We generally think of sounds as impulses that are interpreted by the brain in waking life, but evolutionary instinct has given us the ability to select the sounds we react to during sleep, too. If you call out a person's name while they are in light or REM sleep, they either wake up or incorporate the sound into their dreams and an EEG machine will register changes in their brain patterns. A sleeping mother is able to wake up if her own baby cries, but can ignore another baby's cry even though the sounds are very similar to anyone else. This is even true during deep sleep Stages 3 and 4. Some aspect of us is thus monitoring sounds even while we are deeply asleep. Some sounds can actually enhance our sleep experience. White noise (similar to the hissing of an un-tuned TV) seems to have a soothing effect, as does the sound of the sea even if this is quite loud. Roaring traffic or the clang of a burglar alarm is rather less conducive to sleep! Obviously, the more tired you are, the less likely you are to be disturbed by noise.

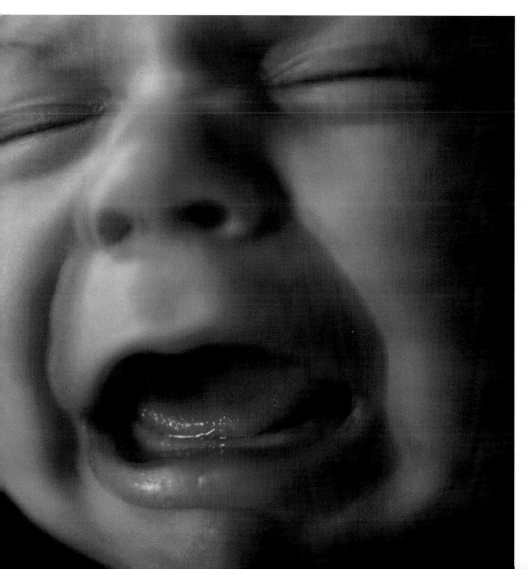

Left: a mother is able to wake up if her own baby cries.

Far right: touching or even breathing in small quantities of certain substances is enough for the allergic person to start sneezing, come up in a rash, have a headache, a runny nose or streaming eyes.

Noise may be an obvious disrupter of sleep, but temperature and humidity should not be overlooked either. Being too hot or cold in bed is sure to either disturb your sleep or prevent you from falling asleep to start with. It is, of course, impossible to say what the ideal temperature for promoting sleep is because we are all different. Some people get very cold at night whereas others actually get uncomfortably hot. Research suggests that a temperature of around 63 degrees F (17 degrees C) is about right for most adults. A baby's bedroom is best kept at a constant 65 degrees F (18 degrees C). Studies have shown that in temperatures of over 74 degrees F (24 degrees C) people wake up more frequently and are more restless during sleep. Most people's body clock makes the body temperature gradually reduce during the night to reach its lowest point at around 4am. Ideally, your central heating controls should reflect this pattern. One problem with central heating, though, is that the air can become very dry and this can irritate the bronchial passages. This can make some people wake up with a dry throat and coughing. A simple bowl of water placed near the heat source should humidify the air and reduce this problem. On the other hand, a room that is too damp can raise stress levels. In very hot weather, it may be tempting to sleep naked with no bed clothes at all. Be warned that if you sweat during the night and have no covering to absorb the moisture, you could easily catch a chill. In hot weather, it is best to sleep under a light sheet made of natural fibres or wear a light night shirt.

AVOIDING ALLERGENS

Allergic reactions take place when the body reacts abnormally to some outside influence. Touching or even breathing in small quantities of certain substances is enough for the allergic person to start sneezing, come up in a rash, have a headache, a runny nose or streaming eyes. Allergic reactions can even cause depression. Breathing is often one of the first things to be affected and this can cause snoring. Doctors can prescribe antihistamine drugs to treat the condition with some success, but prevention is always better than cure. Household dust mites are tiny insects that love warm moist conditions like bedding and mattresses. They can also live in other fabric such as carpets, curtains and upholstery. The droppings of the dust mite are very allergenic so it is best to vacuum the home regularly. Good ventilation will also help deter the dust mite. Many people also have allergic reactions to the chemicals in household cleaning products. If you suffer from these, try to use natural products such as beeswax, baking soda or vinegar instead. Some people are allergic to various animals so pets are best kept out of the bedroom.

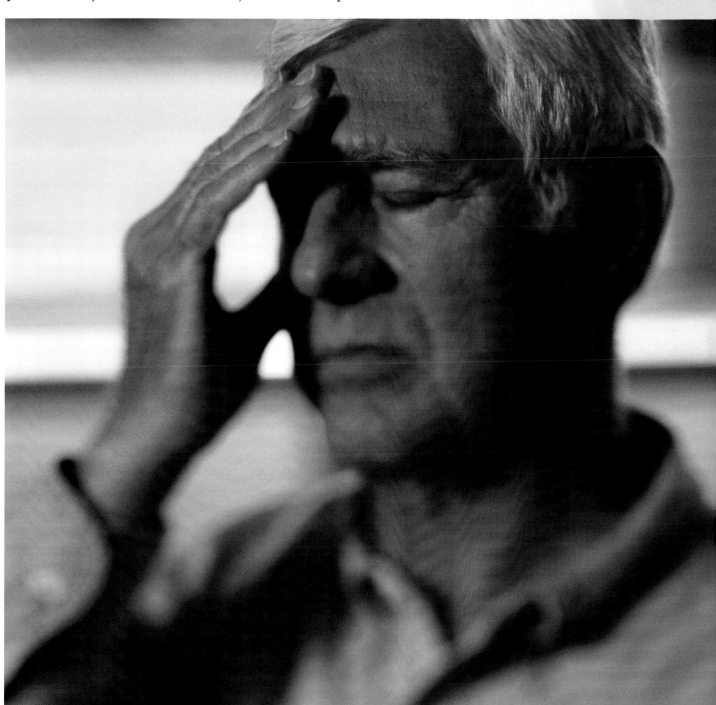

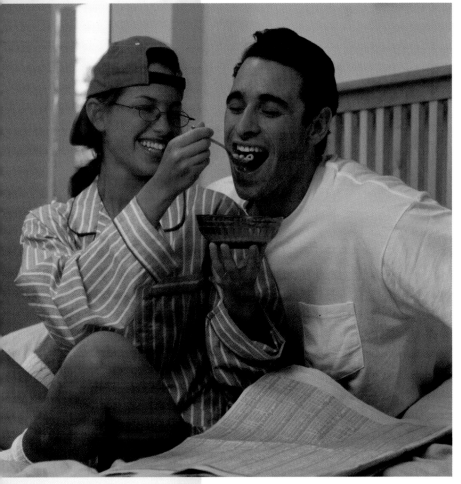

Above: some people's sleep is actually improved by sharing a bed.

sharing a bed. This may partly be because sexual activity before sleep puts us in a relaxed mood. Also many people feel more emotionally secure with a trusted person in close proximity and this may help promote peaceful sleep. People generally move more than ten times per hour during sleep and half of these movements are major changes of body position. Younger couples tend to synchronise their body movements and so do not wake each other up (unless one partner is a loud snorer or insists on reading half the night). However, when couples are separated, each of them moves less during the night. Long-standing couples who have been together for many years seem to move increasingly independently of each other.

SLEEPING WITH A PARTNER

Children usually sleep alone and only begin to share a bed regularly with others after adolescence when they are old enough to start forming intimate relationships. Regularly sleeping with someone else takes some getting used to and often disrupts sleep patterns at first, but evidence suggests that many people's sleep is actually improved by

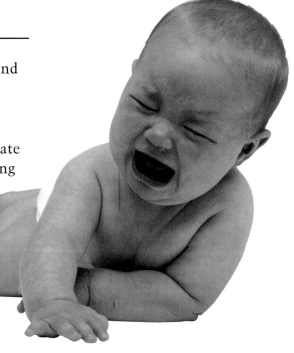

A HEALTHY LIFESTYLE

People are complex beings and we all live on many different levels at the same time. This includes the physical body, through the emotional and mental levels and beyond to the spiritual source from which we all came. In order to stay healthy and function at peak performance in the real world, we need to nourish and develop all these different aspects of our being. Any imbalance in either the physical, emotional or mental body can disturb normal sleeping patterns.

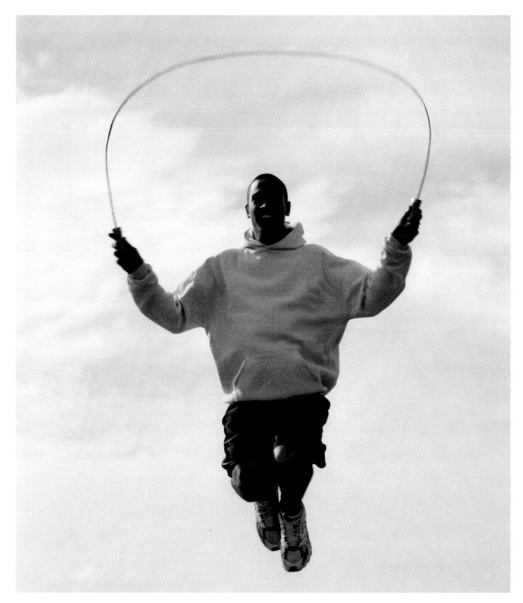

Left: any imbalance in either the physical, emotional or mental body can disturb normal sleeping patterns.

PHYSICAL AND MENTAL HEALTH

The more you look after your overall health, the better your sleep is likely to be. If you go to bed physically healthy, having eaten well several hours before bed, well exercised, emotionally content and free from stress, you will feel relaxed and ready for refreshing sleep. Unfortunately, our modern hectic lifestyle does not make this easy. Work deadlines, city noises and pollution, relationship confusions, and lack of proper exercise all increase our stress levels. This makes it harder to maintain our natural body rhythm. Physical pain will also obviously disrupt normal sleep. We often feel out of balance and all too often try to change our mood and block out our unhappiness artificially by drinking alcohol, smoking, eating junk food or watching TV. Then we stagger into bed more in a state of collapse than ready for natural, regenerative sleep. Under these conditions, it is perhaps not surprising that so many people suffer from poor-quality sleep. It is estimated that as many as 90 per cent of people who suffer from depression and anxiety also complain of sleeping difficulties. Occasional anxiety is often caused by a particular incident such as a relationship break-up or an impending exam and will pass once the problem is resolved. But if longer-term anxiety or depression sets in without any apparent cause, it's time to visit a doctor.

Below: the more you look after your overall health, the better your sleep is likely to be.

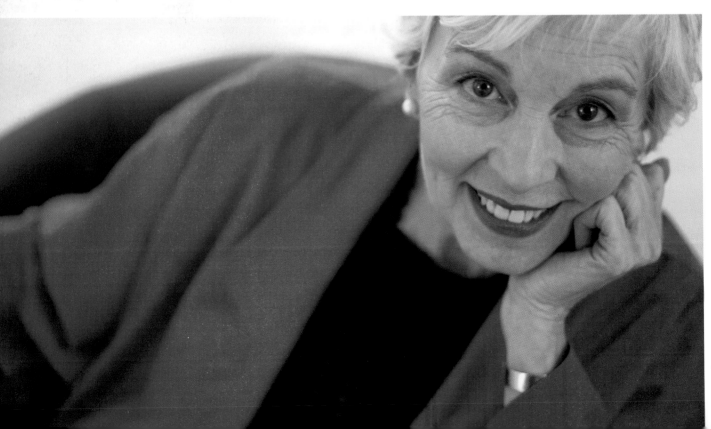

THE BODY CLOCK

Our individual day-to-day experiences may be constantly changing, but we live in a world that has a very regular 24-hour rhythm complete with predictable periods of day and night. Our bodies are naturally attuned to this regular 24-hour cycle or circadian rhythm which is known as our internal "body clock". This internal clock regulates all the systems of the body from digestion and excretion mechanisms through to growth patterns and changes in body temperature etc. All humans and animals have this natural body clock which is situated in the area of the brain known as the suprachiasmatic nucleus. In humans, this area is in the hypothalamus at the base of the brain and close to the optic nerves. This reinforces the connection between the body clock and light and dark. People who stay up at night and consequently sleep during the day are missing much-needed hours of sunlight. They are therefore working against their own body clock that encourages us to go to sleep when it gets dark and wake up when it gets light. Electric lighting confuses the body clock still further. The body clock is influenced by more than just light and dark, however. Experiments have proved that even when volunteers are kept in windowless, permanently lit rooms for weeks on end, they maintained their natural 24-hour body rhythms.

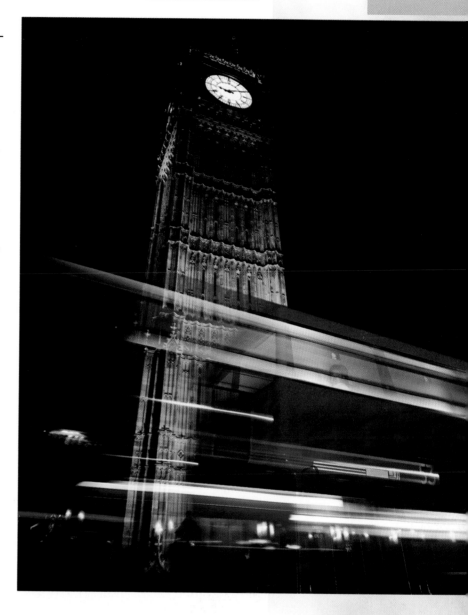

Above: people who stay up at night and consequently sleep during the day are missing much-needed hours of sunlight.

JET LAG

It is, of course, necessary for us to override our body clock from time to time to suit our lifestyle. Long-distance air travel is one such example. After flying through several time zones, we land in a place where our body clock is out of synch with local conditions. This is known a jet lag. We may feel exhausted for several days and bowel movements may be disrupted, but our body will soon adjust to a new 24-hour cycle that is appropriate to local conditions. The best advice for minimising jet lag is to set your watch to the local time of your destination place as soon as you board the plane and try to sleep as much as possible during the flight.

Below: long-distance air travel overrides our body clock.

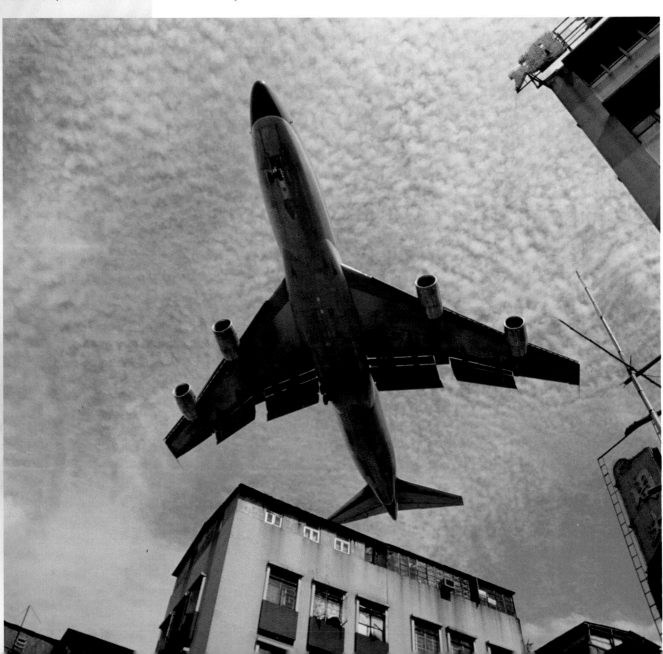

DIET

Whenever we eat, our metabolism speeds up and our body temperature rises as the fuel is absorbed and turned into the energy we need for a healthy, active day. When we are asleep, our body does not need to be topped up with food because we are relatively inactive and are therefore not burning up much fuel. It is best not to eat during the three hours immediately prior to going to bed so that any food in the stomach is already digested and the body can go into rest mode. Some foods are more prone to disrupt sleep than are others. For instance, eating cheese before going to sleep is traditionally thought to produce nightmares.

This is because cheese contains the chemical tyramine which contributes to raising the blood pressure – one of the stress symptoms that occurs during nightmares. On the other hand, a hot, milky nightcap will promote restful sleep. As well as considering our food and drink intake before bed, we should look at our whole diet since the state of our general health will affect sleeping patterns dramatically.

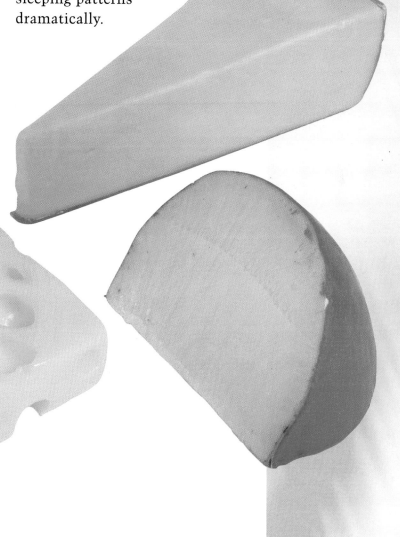

Below: eating cheese before going to sleep is traditionally thought to produce nightmares.

Make sure that whatever your own specific dietary preferences, you are getting the full range of vitamins and minerals. Some studies have indicated that the B complex vitamins are particularly important for promoting good sleep. B vitamins are found in meat, fish, dairy products and seaweed. Remember to use lower-fat cuts if eating meat. Broad beans, potatoes, walnuts and wheat-germ are also high in B vitamins. The mineral magnesium is also thought to aid restful sleep. Bananas, avocados and dark green vegetables are high in magnesium as are nuts and seeds. A low-fat, high-carbohydrate diet has been shown to alleviate depression-related insomnia so eat lots of pasta, bread and potatoes. Try to buy good-quality fresh fruit and vegetables and buy organic food whenever possible, especially when buying meat, since more complex foods can bring more complex problems (as the recent BSE beef crisis has demonstrated). Try also to avoid overly processed foods that may contain a lot of chemicals. Prepare your food well since many general dietary problems such as indigestion and heartburn can ruin a good night's sleep and lower the overall quality of your life. It's your body so value it! Don't underestimate the importance of drinking pure water in maintaining optimum health. It is recommended that each of us should drink 2 litres of water per day. Try not to drink too much just before bedtime, though, or you might find yourself repeatedly visiting the bathroom during the night!

Right: B vitamins are found in meat, fish, dairy products and seaweed.

Far right: people who are slightly heavier sleep better than those who are thin.

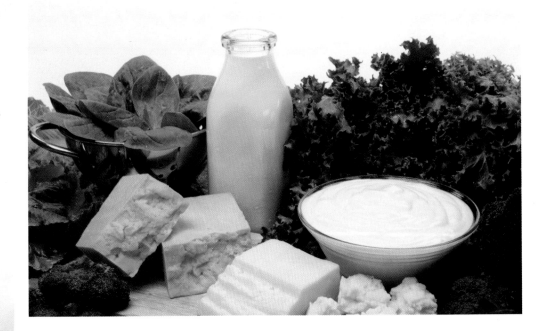

BODY WEIGHT

Being excessively overweight or underweight is clearly a general health issue that affects all areas of life as well as sleep and may need medical attention. However, studies have shown that people who are slightly heavier sleep better than those who are thin. Of course, there may be many reasons for this; happier people who are enjoying life may have healthier appetites. But there is also evidence to suggest that heavier people may have longer sleep cycles which means they spend longer in REM sleep. Overweight people are, however, more prone to snoring. As with all health issues, it is better to avoid extremes so steer clear of crash diets and sudden weight gains.

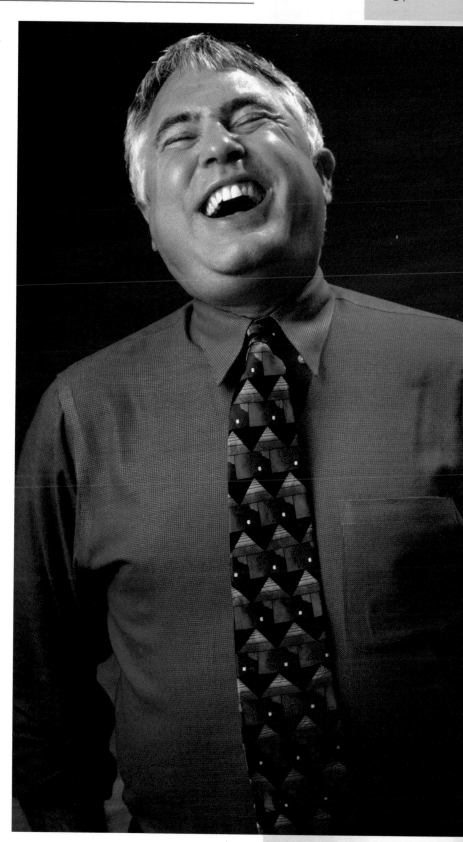

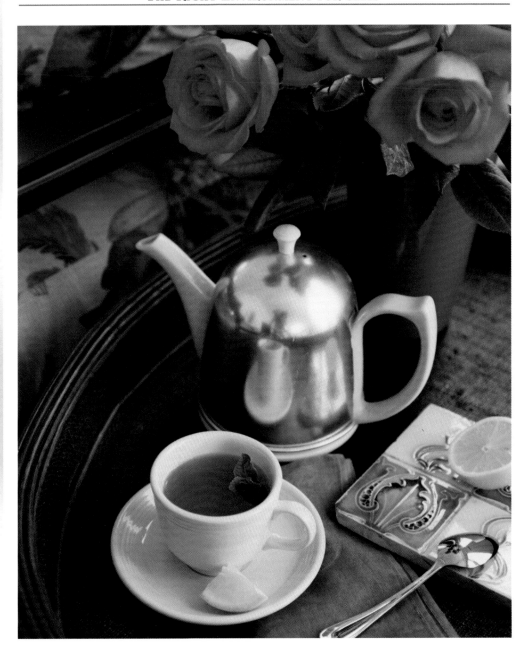

Right: even tea and coffee contain addictive chemical substances.

DRUGS

There are very few of us who could claim to live a totally drug free life. Drugs to many people conjure up visions of crime and debauchery, but even tea and coffee contain addictive chemical substances which, like other drugs, can disrupt normal sleeping patterns. The most widely used drugs that can affect sleep are explored below.

ALCOHOL

Alcohol is widely thought of as a drug that will send us off to sleep – and in small doses this may be true since a glass of wine with dinner or a whisky after work may help us to relax and unwind. Alcohol is, however, a very powerful, addictive and long-lasting stimulant. Even if we fall asleep quickly on going to bed, we are likely to wake up during the night in a hot and sweaty state if alcohol is drunk in large quantities. Excessive alcohol intake also reduces the quality of sleep, even if it does not actually wake us up, since sleep becomes less deep and the time spent in REM sleep is reduced.

Below: a glass of wine with dinner or a whisky after work may help us to relax and unwind.

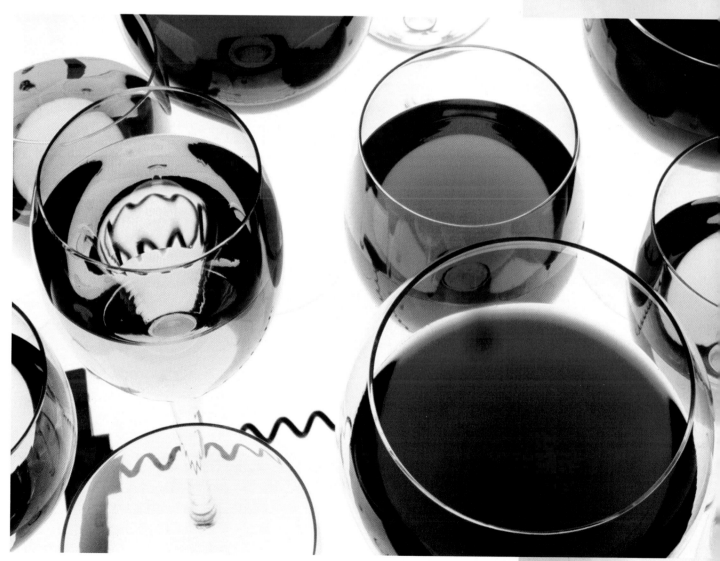

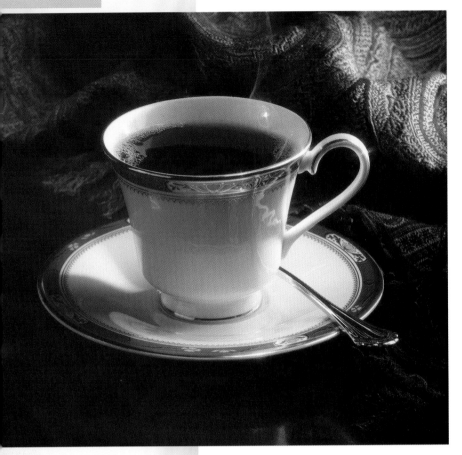

Above: caffeine is a stimulant found in both coffee and tea.

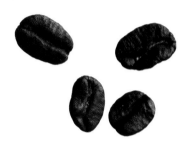

CAFFEINE

Caffeine is a stimulant found in both coffee and tea. It is also present in cola, cocoa and in many over-the-counter cold, flu and pain-relief medications, as well as some prescribed treatments. One of the dangers of caffeine is that it is addictive and the body quickly becomes tolerant of it, so that larger and larger doses are required to feel any effect. Caffeine remains in the body for several hours and has an accumulative effect so that, by night time, there may be a build-up of caffeine in the body that keeps us awake at night. Try to limit your tea and coffee intake by drinking herbal infusions such as camomile and fruit teas instead. If you can't do without the taste of coffee, try the decaffeinated varieties.

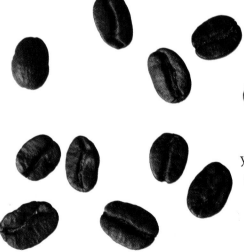

NICOTINE

Tobacco is a plant that contains the highly addictive and poisonous substance, nicotine. Smoking, as we all now know, is a serious health hazard. Anyone suffering from insomnia should have a particular incentive for giving up smoking because nicotine is a stimulant that raises the blood pressure and triggers the release of adrenalin into the blood stream. This will make sleep lighter and more liable to disruption. Also the coughing and other nose and throat problems associated with smoking may contribute to snoring and will certainly affect breathing. Unfortunately, the smoker who wakes up in the night may find a cigarette relaxing. But this feeling of relaxation is only due to the temporary relief of satisfying a craving and will soon pass. Then the stimulating effect of the nicotine will simply keep the smoker awake. At the very least, smokers should ban smoking from the bedroom.

Below: smoking, as we all now know, is a serious health hazard.

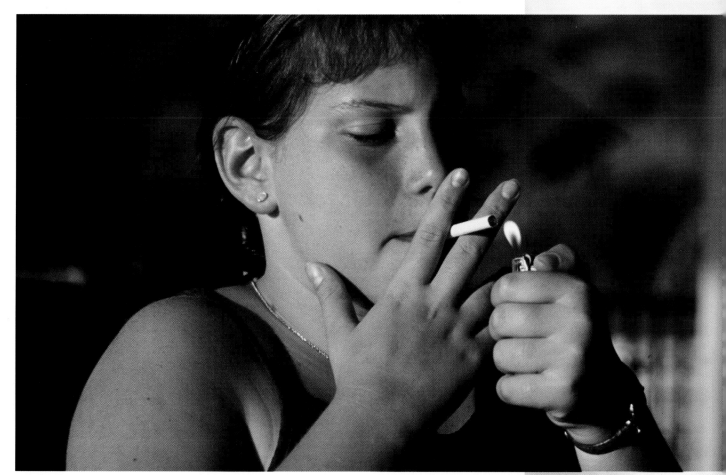

STIMULANTS IN FOOD

Salt is a necessary part of a healthy diet, but our fast-food eating habits mean most of us are eating vastly more salt than is healthy. Salt and salty preservatives such as monosodium glutamate have been linked to insomnia as these stimulate the nerves and can lead to hyperactivity in both children and adults. Children are particularly sensitive to food additives because their immune systems are not yet fully developed. Too much sugar and starch can also create hyperactivity and may therefore lead to insomnia. Processed foods that contain artificial colourings and flavourings and large amounts of salt and sugar should be avoided.

Right: most of us are eating vastly more salt than is healthy.

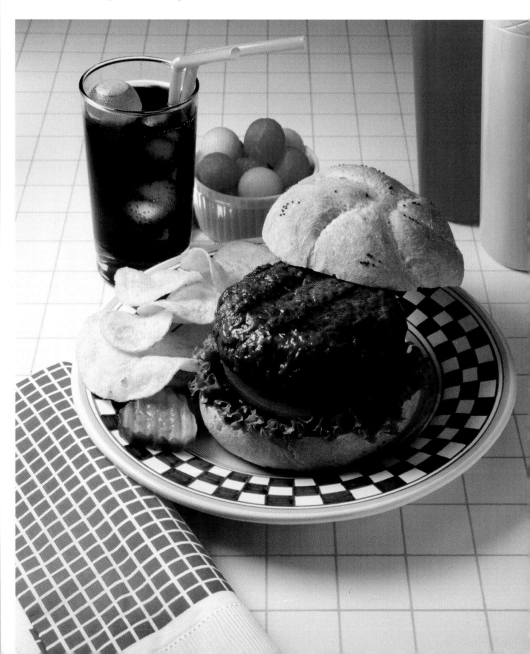

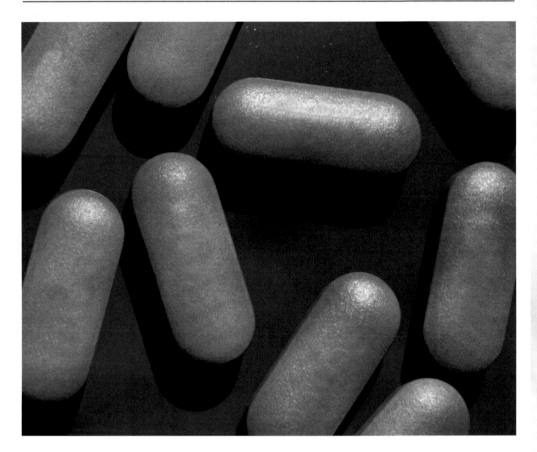

Left: many prescribed drugs can interfere with natural sleep.

PRESCRIBED DRUGS

There are a great many prescribed drugs that may also have the side effect of disrupting sleep. If you find that a prescribed treatment for another condition is affecting your sleep, you should discuss this with your doctor but don't stop taking the medication without your doctor's knowledge. Also, be aware that taking sleeping pills to aid sleep may work for a short time, but can lead to longer-term problems if the body comes to rely on them. Unfortunately, many doctors are still all too ready to prescribe sleeping pills when more natural treatments or even a sympathetic ear are all that is required to help relieve stress and so aid restful sleep. Amongst the many drugs that can interfere with natural sleep are:

Appetite suppressants
Barbiturates
MAO inhibitors
Piracetam
Psychostimulants
Scopolamine
Thyroid hormones
Tranquillisers.

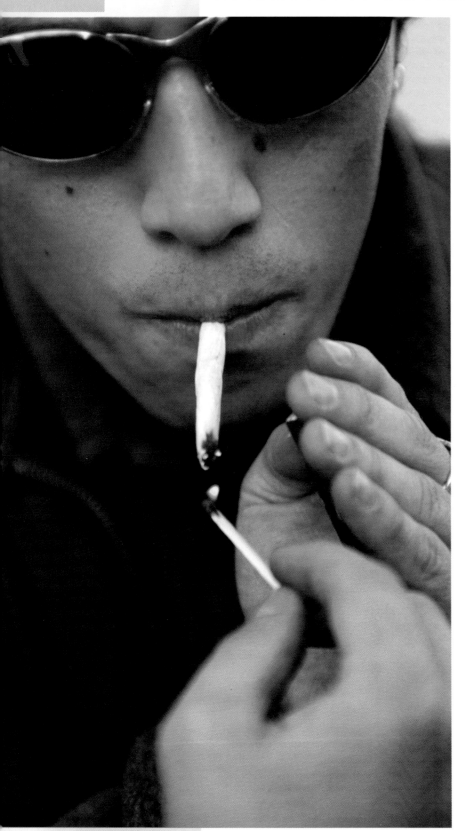

RECREATIONAL DRUGS

Many illegal drugs used recreationally will disrupt normal sleeping patterns both while the drug is being used and during the withdrawal process, in the case of addictive drugs. Some drugs such as amphetamines and cocaine are specifically chosen by people who want to stay awake and alert longer. Cannabis is not physically addictive and is often used in the evening to aid relaxation. However, cannabis is often used with tobacco which is addictive. Cannabis is a mild hallucinogen and all hallucinogens have been shown to change the brain-wave patterns of sleeping subjects. Regular users of cannabis adapt to a new brain-wave pattern during sleep, but this returns to normal once use of the drug has stopped. LSD is another hallucinogen. Opiates are addictive drugs that have historically been used to induce powerful, prophetic dreams in shamanistic cultures around the world. Heroin sold illegally on the street is usually unclean and contaminated with other substances and using this can induce particularly unpleasant visceral nightmares.

EXERCISE

In order to remain healthy, we all need to ensure our physical, emotional and mental bodies are nurtured and maintained. Anyone who takes a long walk by the sea or in the countryside is well aware of how the fresh air, beautiful scenery and physical exertion reduces stress levels, increases the appetite and makes us feel tired but happy and ready for bed in the evening. People who live and work in the open air may have as many problems in their lives as those who have an urban life, but being in touch with nature has a rejuvenating quality not found in city life. People who have sedentary, office-based jobs may feel tired at the end of each day, but this is usually an emotional and mental tiredness and the body may have been inactive all day. On returning home, city dwellers may feel exhausted but with a buzzing mind that just won't quieten down. This can make sleep difficult and encourages us to drink alcohol or watch TV to try to unwind. If you live a sedentary, city life, join a gym and actually use it for 30 minutes every day – you will find the quality of your sleep improves dramatically. Find an activity you enjoy because if you are not enjoying it you will not continue for long. If you are not fit enough for vigorous exercise, try getting off the bus a stop before you usually do and gently walk the rest of the way. Start all new exercise regimes gently and build up as your strength increases. If you have any doubts about your health, talk to your doctor first. But even a small increase in your level of exercise will be enough for you to feel the benefit. Do not take any intense exercise during the couple of hours before your normal bedtime, however, as your body will already be in winding-down mode.

Far left: cannabis is a mild hallucinogen.

Below: join a gym and actually use it for 30 minutes every day.

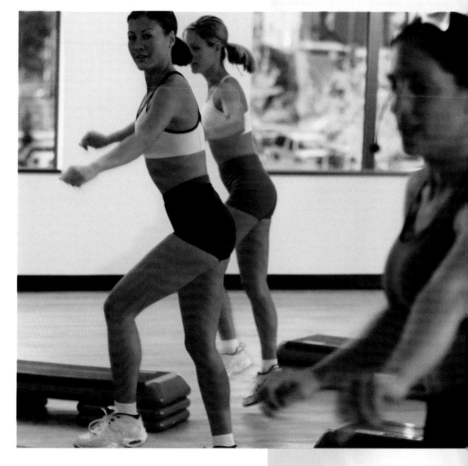

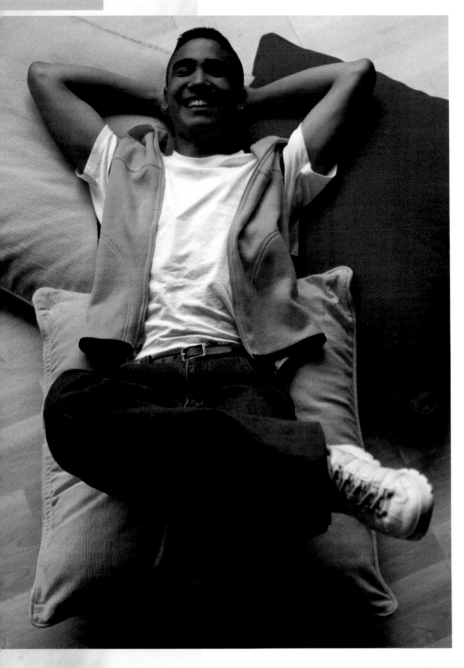

Above: a healthy lifestyle gives rise to a positive frame of mind where we can go to sleep feeling optimistic about the following day to come.

LEARN TO RELAX

In order to drop off to sleep, we have to be relaxed. A good diet, plenty of exercise in the fresh air and healthy, loving relationships will all put us in a positive frame of mind where we can go to sleep feeling optimistic about the following day to come. Worry is one thing guaranteed to keep us awake. It is unrealistic to expect to end each day without a care in the world, but we can learn the self-discipline required to put unresolved issues to one side ready to be dealt with the following day. Here the maxim, "Tomorrow is another day", is particularly relevant. Many people find learning to meditate is useful for relaxing the body and calming the mind. Regular meditation can also help us gain detachment from the immediacy of day-to-day problems. There are many different meditation techniques available with many different philosophies behind them. The sheer quantity of choice and the fear of being lured into a particular religious dogma is enough to make many people suspicious of meditation as a whole. This is understandable, but there are some very simple meditation techniques that anyone can learn which will do no harm and will help you to relax. Firstly, find a place to meditate in which is quiet. Sit comfortably on a cushion on the floor or sit on a straight-backed chair. Rest your hands on your knees or in your lap. Close your eyes, relax and concentrate on breathing through your nose only.

The aim is not to interfere with your breathing in any way, but simply to observe your own natural breathing. It you want a deep breath, then take one – but say to yourself, "Now I'm taking a deep breath". If you want a shallow breath, say to yourself, "Now I'm taking a shallow breath". By keeping focused on your breath, you become less attached to the many thoughts that will inevitably pass though your mind. Whenever a train of thought pops into your head, don't focus on it but simply remind yourself to observe your breath. After 15 minutes of this, you will be surprised at how relaxed you feel. If you continue this practice every day, you may want to increase the time spent meditating gradually to about half an hour per day.

Below: after 15 minutes of meditation, you will be surprised at how relaxed you feel.

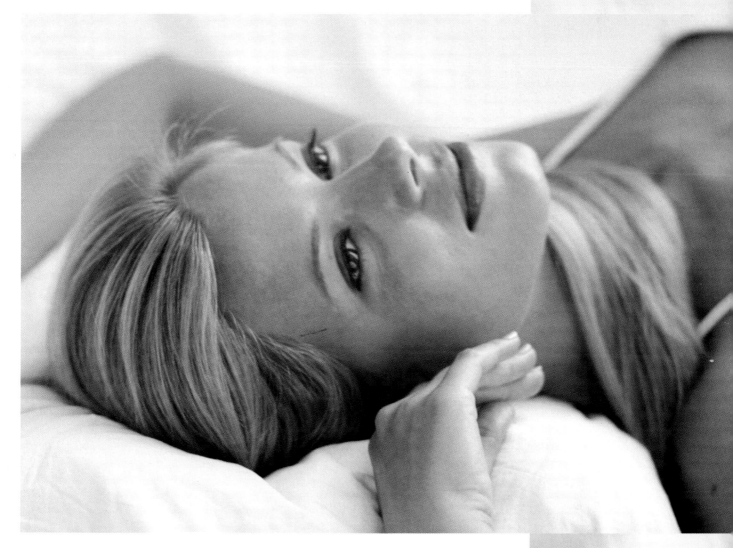

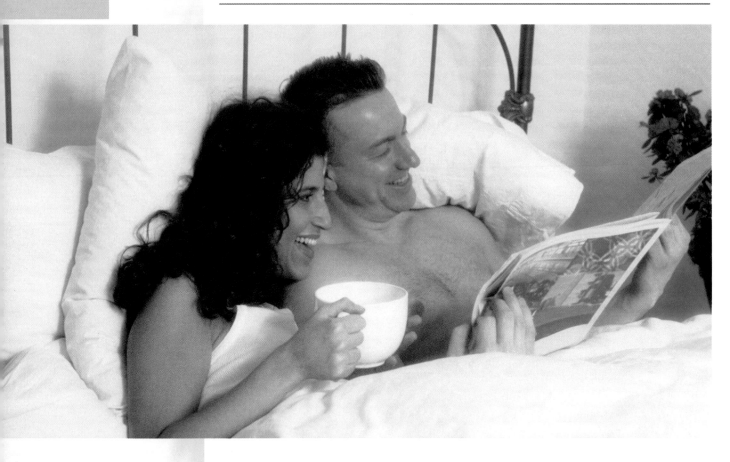

Above: establish a bedtime routine during the couple of hours leading up to bed. This can be as elaborate or simple as you like.

ESTABLISHING A BEDTIME ROUTINE

We discussed earlier how the human body has been instinctively programmed by evolution to work on a 24-hour cycle. This is known as the "body clock". It stands to reason then that the more regular our life habits, the better the body will function. This is very true where bedtime habits are concerned. Essentially, our bodies would prefer to go to sleep and wake up at approximately the same time every day. We may need to sleep more or less on any particular night depending on what has happened to us during the day, but sleeping patterns are also a matter of learned behaviour and habit. For this reason it is good practice to establish a nightly ritual or bedtime routine during the couple of hours leading up to bed so that the body can recognise these cues and begin preparing itself for the impending night's sleep. This can be as elaborate or simple as you like. The important thing is that the bedtime routine should be enjoyable and relaxing.

Pamper yourself and be indulgent! Maybe you would like to soak in a hot bath, perhaps with a few drops of a favourite essential oil. Or maybe there is a particular kind of music you like to listen to. Some people like to have a light snack or have a milky drink shortly before bed. If you eat, keep it light and make sure the food is easy to digest. A cheese and pickle sandwich is perhaps not the best choice! A good way for couples to relax before bed is to give each other a relaxing massage. Skill at massage here is less important than the desire to relax and heal. Massage here may or may not be combined with sexual activity. Sex is a great way to unwind if you have a willing partner and is the perfect way of forgetting the tensions of the day. Another part of your night-time routine may be to lie in bed and read a few chapters of a good novel. Whatever your choice of bedtime rituals, the important thing is that they should be relaxing and as indulgent as you like. The last thing you want is to read through work-related papers or check your business messages. Watching the television is a popular bedtime habit, but is not the most conducive to sleep. Televisions are best kept out of the bedroom altogether, but if you can't do without it don't watch anything that might be disturbing before sleep and don't begin to watch a long movie that will end well after your normal sleep time.

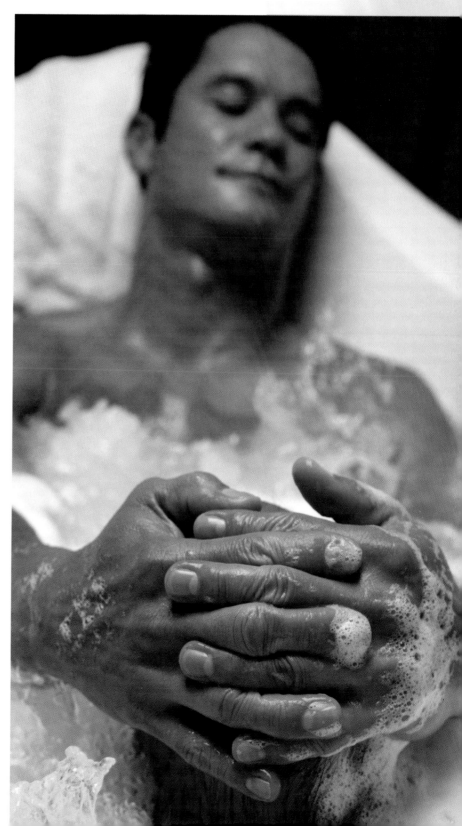

Below: soak in a hot bath, perhaps with a few drops of a favourite essential oil.

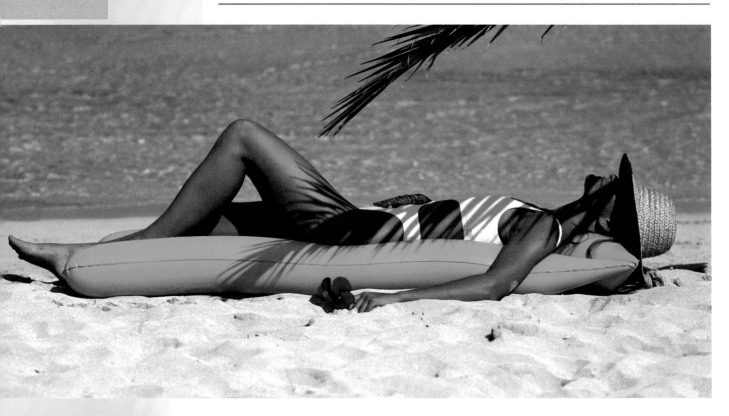

Above: imagine yourself lying on a restful beach.

When you begin to feel sleepy, this is the time to go to bed. If you wait too long, you may start to wake up again. Once in bed, try to let go of all the day's problems. One thing that is guaranteed to keep you awake tossing and turning is feeling angry either with yourself or other people. If there are any tensions between you and your partner, try to talk it out before you attempt to sleep. If sleep still eludes you, you may have success with a simple self-hypnosis technique where you imagine first your feet going to sleep followed by your ankles, then lower legs, body and so on up to your head. Hopefully, you will be asleep well before you reach your head! Alternatively you can imagine yourself lying on a restful beach or in scenic countryside. Breathe slowly and deeply as you absorb the restful environment. If sleep continues to elude you, some people recommend getting up and making a drink or reading a book for a while. Other people find greater success in falling asleep by continuing to lie in bed so as not to break the rhythm. Each person is different so you must find out what works best for you. The following section lists different remedies that people experiencing sleep difficulties can explore.

DRUG TREATMENTS

Sleep problems are very common in our culture. In fact, it is estimated that 40 million people in America alone suffer from some kind of sleeping problem. Given this pressure on the medical profession, it is perhaps not surprising that many doctors are more than willing to prescribe sleeping pills even though many patients may only need a sympathetic listener to help relieve their stress. Unfortunately, taking sleeping pills can actually make matters worse because the body quickly becomes accustomed to them and withdrawing from the pills can be painful and protracted. In fact, withdrawing from an addiction to sleeping pills can be worse than the original problem. Most people fall asleep within an hour of taking sleeping pills, but the sleep that results is not the same as ordinary sleep. Many sleeping pills work by depressing overall brain functions and this can dramatically reduce the time spent in REM sleep. Time spent in deep sleep is also reduced so the sufferer who is still not getting proper sleep may feel they need yet more pills. If you take sleeping pills at all, view them only as a short-term solution to an immediate crisis. Do not use them for longer than two weeks because of the danger of addiction. Long-term use can also lead to severe organ damage. If you are already addicted to sleeping pills, work on gradually reducing your nightly dosage over a period of several weeks under the guidance of your doctor. It is preferable to steer clear of sleeping pills altogether, so instead try some of the gentler but more effective treatments listed below.

Below: if you take sleeping pills at all, view them only as a short-term solution.

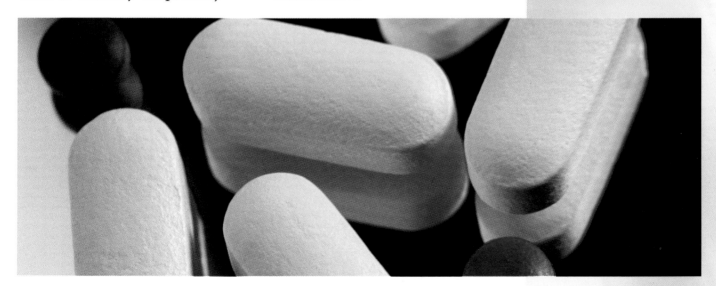

MELATONIN

Melatonin is a sleep hormone that is produced naturally in the brain. During the hours of darkness, melatonin is released by the pineal gland which is situated deep inside the brain. Because of the connection between melatonin and light and dark cycles, it is thought that this hormone controls our natural 24-hour "body clock". Researchers have discovered that melatonin levels in the body increase by as much as 50 per cent in the hours immediately before bedtime and this has led to speculation that additional doses of the hormone may help "reset" the "body clock" and so aid sleep. Melatonin is now being sold as a food supplement, mainly in health food shops in the USA. The treatment is still very experimental, however, and there is some concern about the high doses needed to make any difference to sleep. Pregnant or breast-feeding women are therefore advised to avoid melatonin until further trials are completed. People suffering from depression, heart conditions and those with kidney disease should also avoid melatonin supplements.

Below: melatonin is now being sold as a food supplement, mainly in health food shops in the USA.

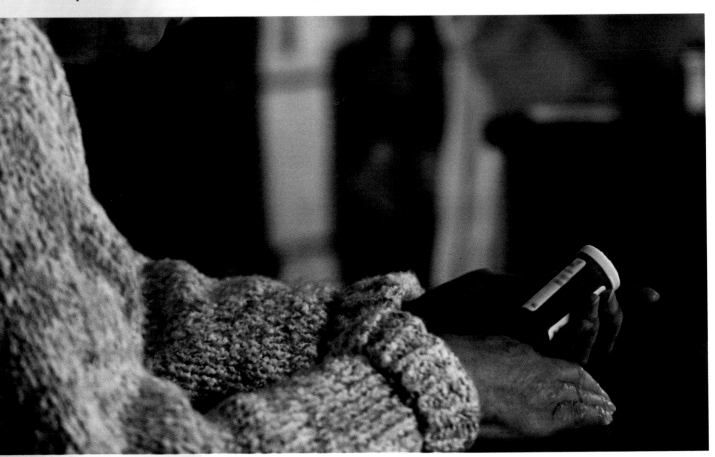

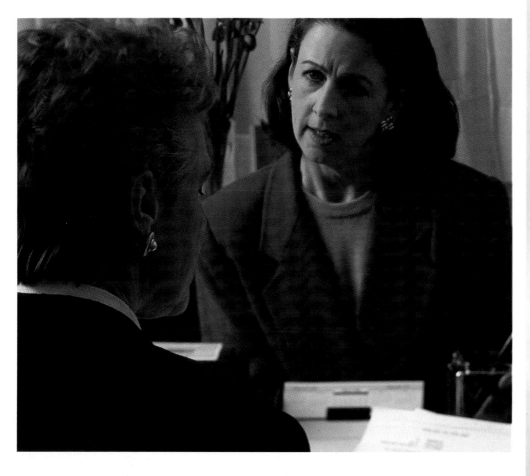

Left: many people who suffer from insomnia would benefit from talking things over with a counsellor.

COUNSELLING

Many people who suffer from insomnia would benefit from talking things over with a counsellor. The first port of call for insomnia sufferers is usually the doctor. But doctors are generally very busy people who do not have time to discuss at length all the emotional and environmental conditions that may well have a bearing on a patient's sleep problems. A counsellor, by contrast, is available to explore all these issues in a relaxed manner. A counsellor may encourage the patient to keep a diary of sleeping patterns. This will help the patient draw parallels between sleeping patterns and the other developments and emotional events in their life. Each counselling session will have a fixed time limit (usually around an hour), but there is often no limit on the number of sessions. The length of overall treatment is usually decided on an ongoing basis during discussions between the counsellor and patient.

Far right: under the guidance of a reputable hypnotherapist, the patient can be given suggestions which become implanted into the subconscious mind that will affect the patient's behaviour long after the actual session.

Below: keep a regular diary of thoughts and feelings.

COGNITIVE BEHAVIOUR THERAPY (CBT)

Cognitive behaviour therapy, or CBT, is an intensive form of therapy that concentrates on trying to help people break through the negative thought patterns that can keep people locked into anxiety and fear. This could be particularly useful for individuals who suffer from insomnia because of anxiety. The treatment consists of a series of up to 20 hour-long sessions where the patient is encouraged by a clinical psychologist to challenge and eventually overcome the negative thoughts, feelings and behavioural patterns that are producing the insomnia. Patients will be asked to keep a regular diary of thoughts and feelings to be discussed at the next session.

HYPNOTHERAPY

The word "hypnosis" is derived from the Greek word Hypnos who was the god of sleep. Hypnosis is a trance-like state somewhere between sleep and waking. In this deeply relaxed state people are very suggestible because the more critical faculties of the mind are suspended. Under the guidance of a reputable hypnotherapist, the patient can be given suggestions which become implanted into the subconscious mind that will affect the patient's behaviour long after the actual session. The therapist may give the patient certain instructions such as, "When you go to bed each night, you will feel very tired and sleep well", or "Your worries will leave you when you go to bed". The theory is that the patient's subconscious mind will remember the instruction and then act on it. The subconscious mind has powerful self-protective mechanisms which will not usually allow the patient to absorb instructions that are against their own moral code, so the dangers of manipulation are small. However, it is best to be cautious when allowing anyone else into your own head, so be sure to pick a reputable hypnotherapist from a recognised organisation.

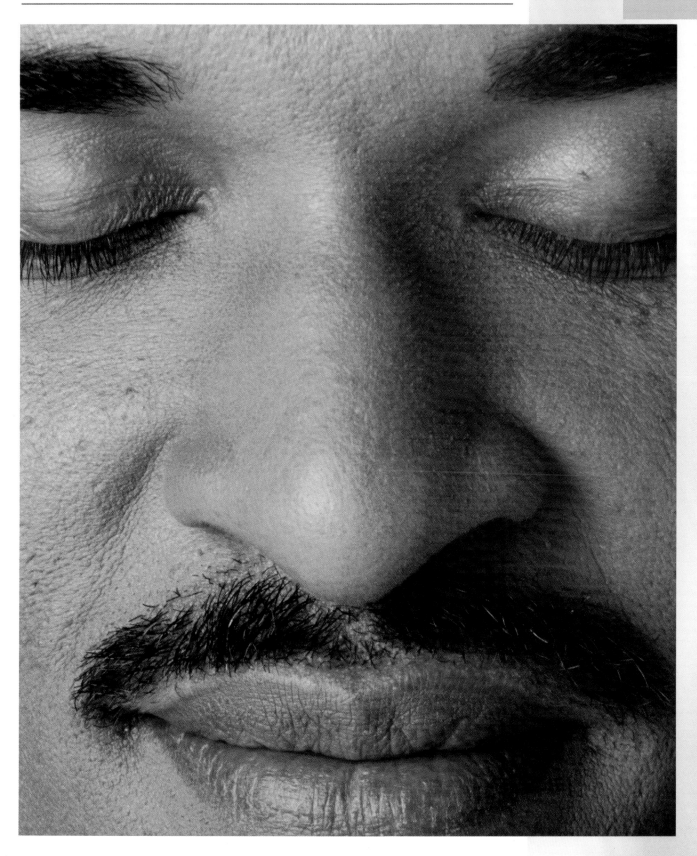

YOGA, TAI CHI

Yoga and T'ai chi are both ancient techniques that have been proven to have a beneficial effect on health and well-being. Both disciplines rely on a set of exercises and gentle movements combined with breathing techniques designed to induce a maximum state of bodily relaxation. The aim in both is to regulate the flow of breath in co-ordination with the movements of the body. This generally has the effect of improving the circulation of the blood around the body due to the increase of oxygen and the release of tension from the muscles. It also tends to improve concentration, build up strength and balance out any extremes in the body's energy. People often feel calmer and more able to relax into sleep. If you're starting as a beginner, yoga or T'ai chi is something you can't really learn on your own. It is best to find a good teacher to start with and learn as part of a group. Once some of the basic techniques have been mastered, a regular practice is essential.

Below: if you're starting as a beginner, yoga or T'ai chi is something you can't really learn on your own.

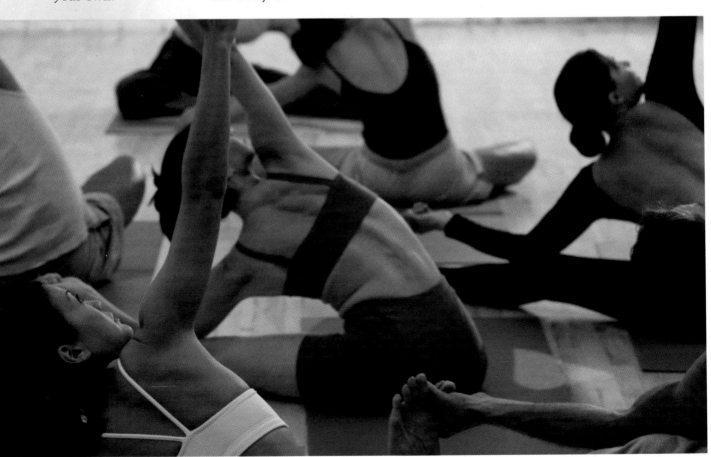

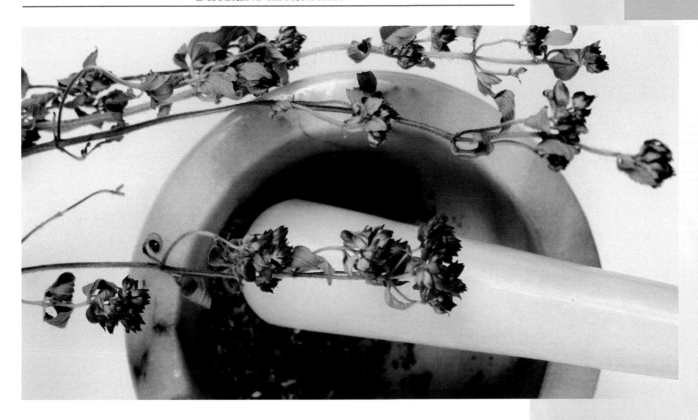

HERBAL REMEDIES

Even from the most ancient times, plants have been utilised for their healing properties. Many of the oldest writings in the world from Sumeria, ancient Egypt and India are devoted to the identification, preparation and uses of plant extracts to treat a wide range of conditions. Most modern drugs are synthetically produced, but even they are often duplicating the substances found in a huge variety of flowers, herbs and trees. Herbalism seeks not only to cure a specific ailment, but rather to treat the whole person by correcting imbalances in the body that can manifest as various health problems including insomnia. Valerian and hops in particular are known to aid sleep. St John's Wort could also be useful especially for those whose insomnia is stress-related. It should not be assumed, however, that because plants are natural, they are automatically safe to take. The substances in some plants can be very powerful and some herbal remedies can be dangerous to people suffering from a variety of medical conditions. Pregnant women and other vulnerable groups should take expert advice from an herbalist before taking herbal remedies.

Above: plant extracts are used to treat a wide range of conditions.

HOMEOPATHY

Below: it is therefore best to seek out a homeopathic practitioner who will prescribe the appropriate treatment.

The basic assumption underlying homeopathy is that "like cures like". Homeopathy was first developed as a therapy in the late 18th century after several years of experimentation by the German doctor, Samuel Hahnemann. The idea is that two similar diseases can't exist in the body at the same time and therefore if a harmless replica disease is introduced into the body, it will stimulate the body's immune system to drive out the harmful disease. Homeopathic remedies are non-chemical and will thus not interfere with any medical treatments. These remedies are readily available in health food shops and should be taken without food or drink or tobacco either 30 minutes before or after. There are many homeopathic treatments which could help insomnia sufferers depending on the cause of the sleep problem. It is therefore best to seek out a homeopathic practitioner who will prescribe the appropriate treatment.

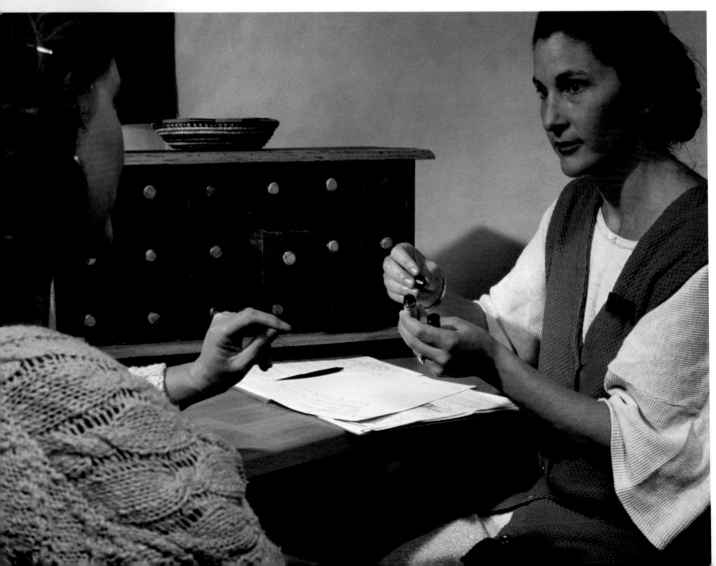

FLOWER REMEDIES

Exponents of flower remedies claim that any disruption in the body's health usually has an underlying emotional or mental difficulty at its core. They claim that particular tinctures from flowers can affect directly and positively both the emotional and mental state of the person taking them, thus freeing the body to heal itself. Though there are now hundreds of flower remedies on the market, hailing from every quarter of the globe, the most well-known are the original 38 essences created in the early 20th century by the British homeopath, Dr Edward Bach. Dr Bach's tinctures are prepared by steeping the petals of particular flowers in spring water and then leaving them to absorb as much sunlight as possible for several hours. The resulting tincture is then mixed with brandy to preserve it. This is administered only a few drops at a time, directly onto the tongue or mixed with a specified amount of still spring water and sipped. In cases of insomnia, where often the causes can be largely due to how we feel or what's going on in our head, Flower Remedies may provide a very gentle solution. There are at least 20 tinctures that are helpful to people suffering sleep abnormalities but all vary in the specifics. For instance, if your sleeping pattern has only temporarily been disrupted due to jet lag or too much work, a few drops of either ylang ylang, dill or banksias robur are appropriate. If you tend to be over-excitable and wound up all the time, Blackeyed Susan, lettuce, verbena, vervain or stock might be a better idea. For those who suffer from nightmares, Green Spider Orchid or Rock Rose may help.

Left: flower remedies may provide a gentle solution to sleep problems.

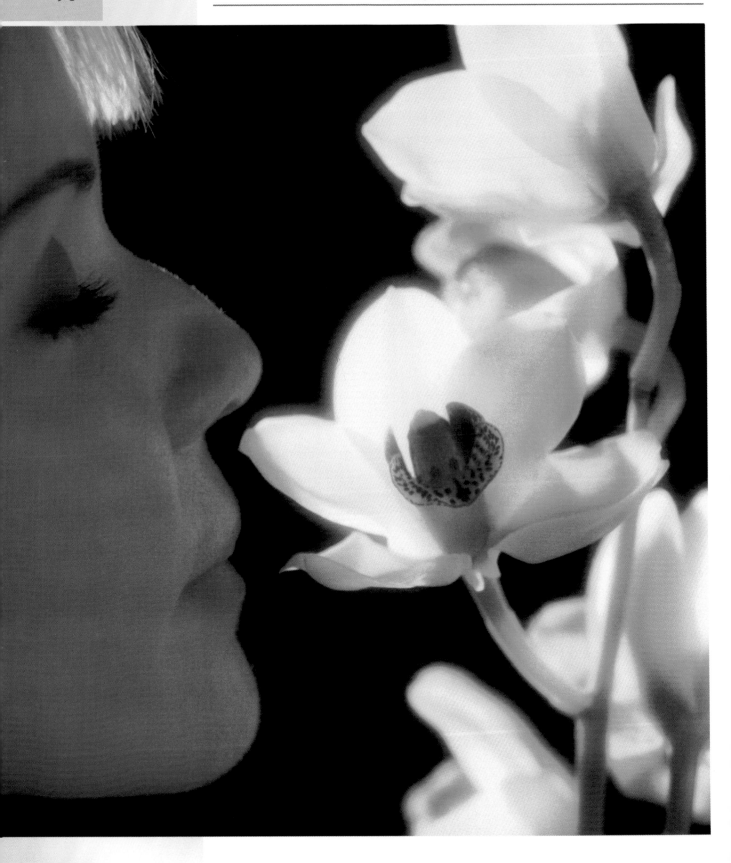

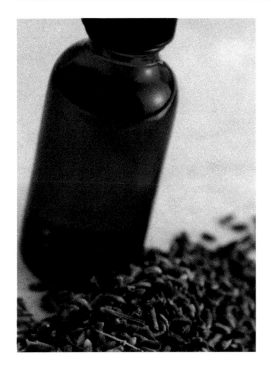

AROMATHERAPY

Aromatherapy involves using essential oils. These are the concentrated extractions of various flowers, leaves, fruits, seeds and roots which can either be inhaled or absorbed through the skin. The aromatherapist will choose one or more oils and blend them together to suit the physical and mental condition of each patient. A few drops of the oils are then mixed with a base oil such as almond or sunflower and used for a full body massage. This can be a particularly effective way of dispersing tension in the body. The oils can also be added to a bath or gently heated in an aromatherapy burner to infuse the air. It must be remembered that essential oils are very concentrated and are too strong to be used on the skin undiluted. They should never be used internally. Also, some oils can be dangerous for people suffering from medical conditions. Children and babies will need much smaller amounts than adults. Essential oils are readily available in health food shops and "new age" shops, but it is best to visit a qualified aromatherapist who will select the right oils for you. Lavender is a very good oil for general relaxation, but there are many more essential oils that are useful for treating the different causes of insomnia.

Left: essential oils are the concentrated extractions of various flowers, leaves, fruits, seeds and roots which can either be inhaled or absorbed through the skin.

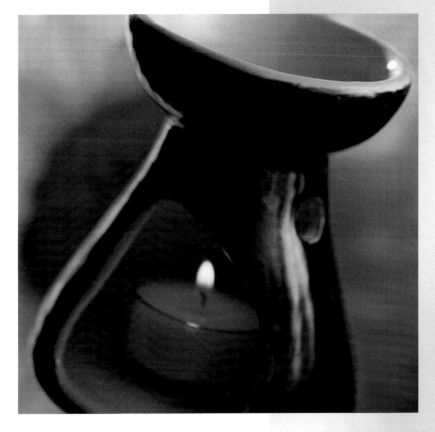

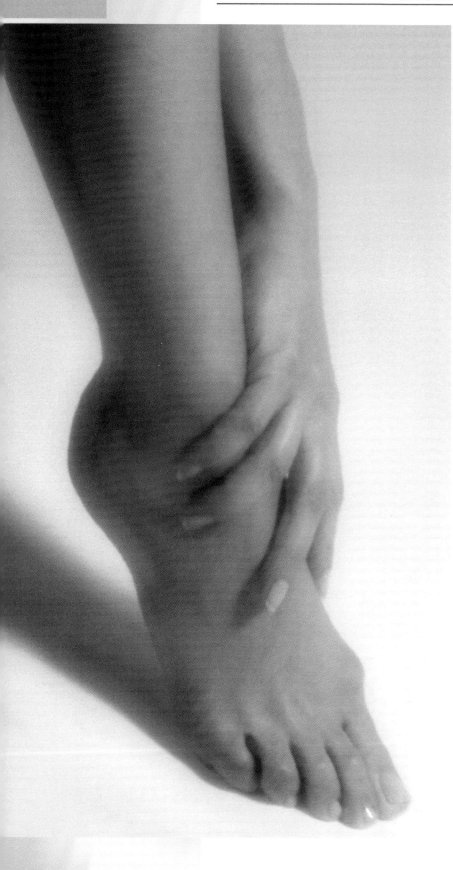

REFLEXOLOGY

Reflexology works on the idea that all the internal organs and areas of the body are reflected in different areas of the feet. The head, for instance, is represented by the big toe and the spine is represented by the inside edge of the foot down to the heel. The reflexologist will massage the patient's feet and when the patient feels pain or sensitivity in a certain area, the practitioner will refer to a chart of the feet which identifies the body area concerned. Tension anywhere in the body will manifest as crystals or resistance in the corresponding part of the foot. This can be gently dispersed over a period of several sessions. No specific trials have been conducted into reflexology and insomnia, but many people feel very relaxed after a treatment and sleep unusually well afterwards. Gently massaging your own feet can be very beneficial too. Pregnant woman or those receiving medical treatment should not have reflexology.

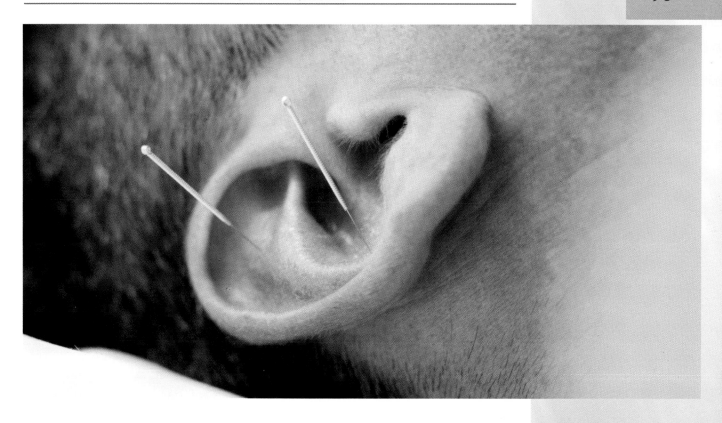

ACUPUNCTURE

The ancient science of acupuncture has been used for thousands of years in China to treat a vast range of medical conditions. The practice consists of inserting fine needless into precisely chosen areas of the body. The philosophy behind acupuncture is that the whole body contains many invisible pathways known as meridians through which an invisible, universal energy known as Qi (pronounced "che") flows. Qi is created by the dynamic interplay of the opposite but complimentary forces of "yin" and "yang", negative and positive energy. Optimum health requires balancing the yin and yang forces in the body. Acupuncture needles are inserted into meridian lines to unblock areas where the Qi energy has either become stuck or is moving too quickly. No definitive trials have been carried out to prove the benefit of acupuncture to insomnia sufferers, but acupuncture can help alleviate many medical conditions if conducted by an experienced acupuncturist. As with all treatments, make sure you see a qualified practitioner so there are no health risks from unclean needles, for instance.

Above: acupuncture consists of inserting fine needless into precisely chosen areas of the body.

Far left: the reflexologist will massage the patient's feet.

INDEX

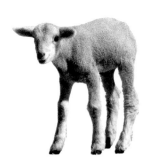

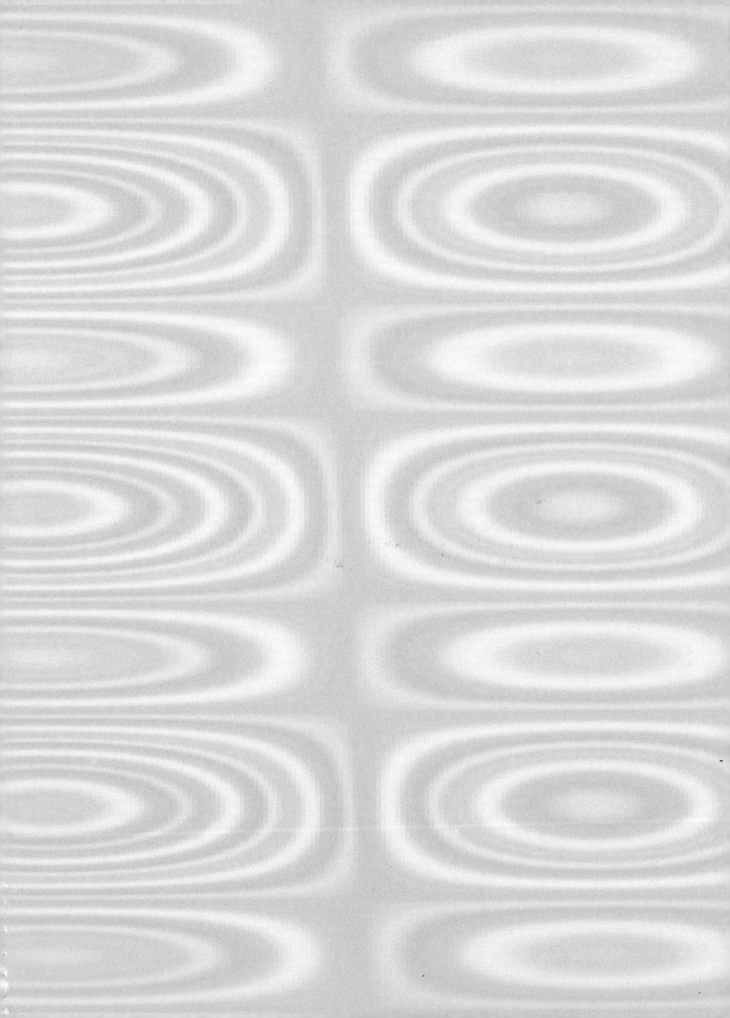